UNDER ONE SKY

**Intimate Encounters with Moms and Babies
by a Breastfeeding Consultant and Nurse**

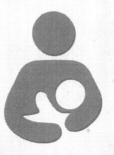

CHRIS AUER

PRAECLARUS PRESS, LLC

WWW.PRAECLARUSPRESS.COM

Praeclarus Press, LLC

2504 Sweetgum Lane

Amarillo, Texas 79124 USA

806-367-9950

www.PraeclarusPress.com

DISCLAIMER

The information contained in this publication is advisory only and is not intended to replace sound clinical judgment or individualized patient care. The author disclaims all warranties, whether expressed or implied, including any warranty as the quality, accuracy, safety, or suitability of this information for any particular purpose.

ISBN: 978-1-946665-12-6

©2018 Chris Auer. All rights reserved.

Cover Design: Ken Tackett

Developmental Editing: Kathleen Kendall-Tackett

Copy Editing: Chris Tackett

Layout & Formatting: Nelly Murariu

CONTENTS

Acknowledgements

The author would like to thank Deb Johnsen who influenced her decision to become a nurse, that being the first step toward her work in Pediatric Intensive Care, then Maternity and the Newborn Intensive Care at the University of Cincinnati Medical Center. The next trajectory into Lactation began by simply observing friends, Susan Vogel and Linda Meyer, nurse their firstborns. It continued with the comradery of Susan Mueller, herself a lactation consultant, but also close friend and neighbor. In addition, she would like to acknowledge the guidance and support of her writing group, particularly poet and teacher Valerie Chronis Bickett (*Our Lives with Words*) and poet Lynn Robbins. A deep debt of gratitude is owed Trudelle Thomas for her invaluable contribution to this manuscript. This book would not have come to fruition without the knowledgeable editing and guidance of the staff of Praeclarus Press. Thank you Kathleen Kendall-Tackett and Ken Tackett. Connecting with these individuals were seemingly small events but created a tectonic shift in Chris' personal journey.

Before the real tectonic shift, creating the continents we know today, we were one land mass. What a difference it would make if we were mindful of our unity, despite oceans (of difference) between us. This book is dedicated to that hope and to my true companion, Ron, who shares it with me.

Under One Sky,
There's a baby's cry.
Under one sky,
A mother's lullaby,
Under one sky we are all a part of everything.

Musical Excerpt, *Under One Sky* by Chris Barton

Introduction

*I'm embarrassed to be doing so
much beautiful work. Seldom has a
human being been so fortunate...*

ALBERT SCHWEITZER

This book took shape due to a growing appreciation for the amazing diversity I've encountered during my years as a breastfeeding consultant and nurse at the University of Cincinnati Medical Center. The stories were born from many moments spent primarily with mothers—but also fathers, and certainly babies—at a significant time in their lives. These precious liminal moments surrounding birth have positioned me at the threshold of encounters with something holy. Of this, I am certain. Have you been privy to encounters like this too and wept the tears they invoke? I hope so. This book is dedicated to those families who welcomed me into a moment in their life journey.

By definition, this liminal space allows for uniting experiences, where the barriers of difference evaporate, only to leave those involved on common (sacred) ground. While they came from different backgrounds, life experiences, customs, and countries, the families reminded me daily that parenthood is a great equalizer. We have common hopes and dreams for our young. I invite you into their stories and into our unitive experiences. They're yours for the taking. We seem to need unity now more than ever. I hope their stories give you pause to rethink the ways you are connected to others who are different than yourself.

I've cared for thousands of women from over 77 countries while working in the maternity field, and have worked for the last 25 years in lactation. The sheer number of patients make most of them fade in memory. Those I do recall are unique, yet at times, they represent many others. In one way or another, they've all left an indelible imprint within me. From the Nepali mother who, like many first-time mothers, innocently asked her questions surrounding care of a newborn, to the epic journey of certain mothers from Congo and Eretria, some of whom gave birth to previous children while in a refugee camp or were simply stuck in the camps for years. Resilience after adversity is both humbling and inspiring to witness.

I've written over 100 stories. Each set of stories comprise a chapter in a particular category. I begin with stories of those who were foreign-born and follow with stories of some of our wonderful hospital interpreters. Among the chapters are stories about staff members (lactation consultants, neonatologists, nurses) that have inspired me and given me valuable insights. The families know better than me that they are the recipients of the knowledge, dedication, and humanity of these men and women whom I proudly call colleagues. There is a chapter about the American-born mothers on the Mother-Baby unit, some of our friendships go back nearly 20 years. I've included chapters dedicated to teens and to mothers with a history of drug use. Working in a teaching hospital, I have included stories of medical and lactation interns. There is a chapter of stories about encounters with mothers after they've been discharged as well as a chapter about loss. Besides a chapter dedicated to phone calls and health fairs, I've included a short chapter on the use of donor milk.

The Newborn Intensive Care Unit (NICU) has the largest number of staff. I've included some of their personal stories and, of course, the stories of those babies and families under their care. Because our hospital is a tertiary care center, we have many mothers in critical condition and who have complex diagnosis well before their pregnancies. This leads to consults in the adult Intensive Care (ICU). Some of these encounters involved mothers who've had an emergency admission that occurred well past the newborn stage. While a few stories are tragic, many are simply encounters of human interest that have occurred surrounding birth. There are memories that left me smiling when they occurred, as well as upon recollection. I hope they leave you smiling too. They have their own chapter. I would be remiss if I did not include the breastfeeding stories that came from my neighborhood and my own family. They were part of my growth as a nurse and lactation consultant, as well as mother and grandmother.

For the most part, I've written in narrative form, but some stories seemed more suited to poetry. When appropriate, I've changed patient names and dates to protect privacy; my writing has been vetted with care to comply with the Health Insurance Portability and Accountability Act (HIPPA). Still, the essence of each story is true. The core of each conversation is accurate, though in a few cases the words spoken aren't verbatim. The stories easiest to write were those that I'd jotted notes about right after the encounter. I omitted the few stories that I couldn't corroborate.

Little did I know that a career as a lactation consultant would capture me and provide so much insight into motherhood and how each mother is shaped by her culture and history—her larger story (and, at times, these stories were larger than life). Appreciation for others who are different than us takes a certain open receptivity that I have only grown into over time. It's certainly critical when caring for patients, but also essential when we live in the midst of so much diversity.

I have learned by trial and error what is helpful, what is not, when companioning mothers and fathers, and am most grateful for the opportunity to be taught by them. Personally, this career has given me immense meaning, growth, and gratification. I hope that the stories I share will resonate and establish common ground among us, no matter how different we may be.

CHRIS AUER

Cincinnati, Ohio
November, 2017
christineauer952@gmail.com

Chapter 1

MEMORIES

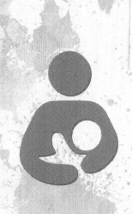

Under One Sky

CHRIS AUER

multi-lingual, illiterate,
lip-readers, signers,
attentive to hunger cues
responsive to babies' needs.

Nepali, Nicaraguan, Nigerian,
Sudanese, Zimbabwean, Welsh,
Mauritanian, Kuwaiti, Uzbek,
Iraqi and Puerto Rican.

refugee, citizen,
naturalized, undocumented,
intuitive knowing –
mothers' milk heals.

Australian, American, Afghan,
Guatemalan, English, Canadian,

Honduran, Ethiopian, Syrian,
Congolese and Vietnamese.

stay at home,
live alone,
work at home,
work-away moms.

South Korean, Senegalese, Sudanese,
German, Bosnian, Salvadoran,
French, Turk, Irish,
Filipino and Saudi.

coffee, peach,
olive, cinnamon,
charcoal, ivory,
chestnut, cream.

Bolivian, Bangladeshi, Burmese,
Ghanaian, Italian, Iranian,
Libyan, Mexican, Burundian,
Rwandan and Sierra Leonean.

impoverished, wealthy,
lowest caste, highest,
no cost mother's milk –
saving lives.

Colombian, Cuban, Costa Rican,
Eritrean, Venezuelan, Pakistani,
Argentinian, Lithuanian, Algerian,
Palestinian and Israeli.

breasts freely exposed,
hijab scarf-covered heads,

sleep deprived,
deferred needs.

Moroccan, Malaysian, Malian,
Croatian, Serbian, Czech,
Romanian, Spaniard, Indian,
Chinese and Somali.

joyful, pensive,
rocking–firstborn, lastborn,
healthy full-term,
sick preterm.

Japanese, Jamaican, Jordanian,
Russian, Pole, Thai,
Kenyan, Cameroonian, Brazilian,
Dutch and Sri Lankan.

skin-to-skin,
bonding,
worlds apart,
under one sky.

1960 Early Memories

We persist and linger longer than we think,
leaving traces of ourselves wherever we go.

DINAW MENGESTU

HOW TO READ THE AIR

When I was 6, we welcomed Geraldine into our humble home. She was a 19-year-old African American neighbor that mom had hired to babysit me, my sister, and younger brother when my mom began full-time work to help make ends meet. Prior to this, mom had bartered childcare for room and board. At that time, we had a young lady from a rural community live with us while she attended a local beauty school. She and I grew especially close. There is a bond that comes from the first experience of being chosen. This mattered. I think it mattered a lot, actually. Geraldine made up an imaginary friend that only she and I could see. She dubbed him our *little purple friend.* My siblings were left out of our imaginary play, mostly because they said they didn't see anything in Geraldine's hand. I knew good and well there was no little purple friend. But when I was with Geraldine, and she held him in her hand and carried on a conversation among the three of us, I was taken in and it was real to me, at least in the Velveteen Rabbit real kind of way. Did our friendship set my internal hardware to a stance of trust? I only know that many years later my muscle memory drew upon memories of Geraldine, which led me *toward* those different from me.

By the age of 8, we moved to Amelia Avenue, immediately across the street from my grandparents. It was pure gift having them so close. If I joined them for a meal, sometimes Flori was at the table too. Flori was a middle-aged Mexican gentleman who worked with my grandpa. He was soft-spoken, gentle, and easy-going. There was nothing substantial to our talks: something about the yard, my grandparents, or my day. Even as a child, I sensed the ease of the interchange between Flori and my adult family members, and it made me comfortable in the presence of someone whose second language was English. I've come to believe that this hardwiring runs deep, allowing me to be at ease connecting to others, even when there is a language barrier.

A few times per year, grandma hired a Hungarian housekeeper named Irma. One day, Irma told me with complete nonchalance that she was a gypsy. I took that to mean nomad and conjured up pictures of her wandering Europe before setting sail for America. I knew nothing else of this culture, but had a naïve sense of its romance. Irma's accent was heavy and she never appeared to mind my visits to pester her as she cleaned. I found it fascinating when she revealed that she told fortunes using cards. I begged her to tell my fortune, but this request always fell on deaf ears. She never seemed exasperated with the questions of a curious youngster.

It may have been in the cards. During my formative childhood years, close contact with these three individuals were instrumental in gravitating me toward a diverse population in my work as a lactation consultant. I hope I have succeeded most days in helping people know that their inherent value is not based on culture, race, religion, gender, or even successful breastfeeding. It just is.

Chapter Two

AROUND THE WORLD ON THE MOTHER–BABY UNIT

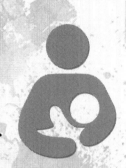

Border Crossings in Africa

Sometimes in the middle of nothing,
hope breaks through and gives you something.

ETHIOPIAN WOMAN,
OXFAM INTERNATIONAL WEBSITE (2016)

I knock and someone from within answers, "Yes?" The scene I come upon is quiet. The woman sits upright in bed, demure expression, cradling her newborn. A man is on the couch with a young boy who's quietly reading a book in an unfamiliar language.

"Zahra," I say slowly as I look at the mother's chart and then at her, "What a beautiful name." I tell them my name, touch her shoulder, and rub the baby's cheek as I speak, while the mother smiles in silence.

Before I pick up the interpreter phone, her husband stops me and tells me he wants to do the translating. This isn't our policy, but he looks at me so intent that I reply back, "Okay, let's just see how it goes."

The question of her previous breastfeeding experience prompts a deluge of information related to their survival instead. He sits on the very edge of the couch, thin, worn face, and speaks in earnest. They are from the small country of Eritrea, and I acknowledge that I know it was previously part of Ethiopia and that it's situated off of Ethiopia's northeast border. He is pleased that I know this, smiling and nodding his head.

He continues speaking while she brushes the black swirls of her daughter's hair with her fingertips. He was in the military for far too many years because conscription is mandatory and the government has the right to keep you indefinitely. To get out, he had to leave the country, escaping by boat 6 years prior. He arrived on the European island of Malta, just 50 miles south of Italy. Meanwhile, Zahra, their then 3-year-old son and 9-year-old daughter, left Eritrea as well, fearing there would be retaliation on the family for his desertion. His family crossed both the northern and southern borders of Ethiopia to arrive in Dadaab, the world's largest refugee camp, situated in the desert of northern Kenya. I picture her, a little less worn than she is today, son strapped to her back with colorful clothe, daughter's small hand in hers. He tells me that the bribes to cross through Ethiopia can be as staggeringly high as $10,000 U.S. dollars. These are the prices people pay to escape to a refugee camp, mind you, not exactly freedom. This particular camp houses three generations of refugees. She and the children were there for 3 years.

After a period of time in Malta, he connected with an agency similar to the Red Cross, though, as we talk, he can't recall its name. They not only secured him a flight to America, but they helped get his family out of the refugee camp, to a different location. When the time came, they flew out of the country to the U.S. He's wide-eyed when he tells me that it cost $4,500 U.S. dollars for their three tickets to Cincinnati 10 months prior to today. It takes little calculating to know that she was pregnant within the month. I'm not asking for assurance, yet he tells me that once he's established with a job in Cincinnati, and his wife has recuperated from the birth and is learning English, he will begin to repay the debt.

He's thanking me now for no specified reason. I've been speechless through this retelling. At some point, I've sat down on the bed, holding his wife's hand throughout. The energy that flows from her to me seems like a momentary jolt from the shock of touching a charged door knob. It's not my imagination, and it's equally unexpected as the story I've just heard. She is smiling, and her drooping ovoid eyes remain serene. I surmise she knows he has been telling their story. How do you communicate admiration and awe without words?

The baby, who's been lying peacefully in the cradle of her arm, stirs briefly. She doesn't hesitate. In one singular movement, she opens her gown, slides the edges of her hair off to the side, and latches him on to her breast, then looks up at me and smiles.

Postscript

According to Human Rights Watch, Eritrea is considered to have one of the worst human rights records in the world. "To charity workers, Dadaab Refugee Camp is a humanitarian crisis; to the Kenyan government it is a *Nursery for Terrorists*, to the Western media, a dangerous No-go area; but to its half a million residents, their last resort."–Ben Rawlence, *City of Thorns*

The Pakistani Muslim and the Jewish Twins He Saved

This world is full of conflicts and full
of things that cannot be reconciled. But there
are moments when we can...reconcile and
embrace the whole mess, and
that's what I call "Hallelujah."

LEONARD COHEN

Days after 9/11, I asked to have lunch with our medical director of Obstetrics. Doctor Tariq Siddiqi is a Pakistani Muslim. He is also a renowned perinatologist whose focus is complicated, high-risk pregnancies. He graciously responded to my inquiries about his faith, which I so wanted to understand after the tragic events in New York, Washington, and Pennsylvania. During lunch, he quotes a couple sayings attributed to Mohammed. One that I recall is that, "Paradise rests at the feet of the mother." It reminds me of a bumper sticker I'd seen years earlier that said if grandmothers ran the country there would be no more war. At least, I hope, a few less. I heard no religious or political inference nor animosity from my colleague that day. Dr. Siddiqi is always a calming presence to his patients, and a confident, but humble clinician. He was that same calming presence with me, as he talked about how fast-growing Islam is, of late, in the U.S. I had no idea. When I asked if he could speculate on why, he only mentions that his religion has a rich experience in community as extended family. He thought this, in particular, appealed to some.

As he spoke, my mind drifts back to something that occurred a few years prior. Four years earlier, a Jewish couple pregnant with identical twins came into this physician's life. When the mother's abdomen grew at an abnormally fast pace, the couple was referred to Dr. Siddiqi. He promptly diagnosed Twin-to-Twin Transfusion, a potentially fatal syndrome for identical twins. It develops when the blood supply they are sharing with one placenta becomes unevenly distributed between the twins. The "donor twin" becomes growth restricted, and the baby floats in decreasing amounts of amniotic fluid while the "recipient twin" is deluged with a blood supply that stresses the heart. Non-treatment is 100% fatal for one or both fetuses. However, treatment is not without risk. His intervention saved both babies' lives. Guided by ultrasound, he inserted a needle into the larger amniotic sac to drain off excess fluid. In their case, he performed this procedure five different times. The interventions worked for Gabriel and Elijah.

I met the couple after the preterm births of their sons, and watched as their babies' status went from guarded to stable. They were 6 weeks early. It's routine that once the NICU staff learn the name of a baby, someone calligraphies their name, adds a little art work onto a 3-by-5 card and attaches it to the incubator. I was touched when I saw that the parents had chosen Dr. Siddiqi's first name as the middle name for both Gabriel and Elijah. On day of life 8, it was Dr. Siddiqi who performed the circumcisions, the ceremonial bris, while their rabbi officiated. Again, I admired the intentionality of the parents. They had a relatively brief 20-day stay, and were discharged knowing the rudiments of how to breastfeed. Each time I worked with mom, the focus was always on latch. We never discussed the naming of their babies.

Their story was written up in our local *Enquirer* newspaper. Dr. Siddiqi was quoted as saying that if religion is practiced the way it is preached, there is no faith that says to harm others. The mother said their religious view was that God is God, specific faith was immaterial.

This couple chose to make a very public tribute, and ultimately a show of solidarity, with a Muslim, when they named their sons Tariq. This encounters, imbued with its unique sweetness, left me with feelings of connectedness to those of other faiths.

The Filipino's Insistence
on a Massage

*I've learned that every day you should reach
out and touch someone.*

MAYA ANGELOU

I am on-call tonight, hoping I'm not needed. It's been a long day caring for my granddaughter, then tutoring kindergarteners at an urban school, but the phone rings and there are a few mothers and babies to check on. I arrive on the unit and speak first to a nurse in L & D. She tells me about a mom she recently transferred to the maternity side.

"She pushed quite a while. They used a vacuum, but only very briefly. I tried to help with latch during skin-to-skin time, but the baby seemed in a daze. Mom had lots of colostrum and I helped her just drip it into the baby's mouth."

"What time was the birth?" I asked with nonchalance, as I glanced over the census.

"Nine. Oh, she also had a tubal, and it took quite a while to send a piece of the tube to the lab to confirm it was her tube, due to adhesions around the area, and we had to keep her over here all day. Actually, we tried the breastfeeding three times total while she was over here. With the way her milk dripped, I'd say she got three feedings in, even though she never latched," she says with a smile of satisfaction.

I go to the unit and see this mom first. She is there with
the nurse, her own mother, and her baby, named Hope. It's
hard for mom to sit up, so I ask if she can lean off to the side,
perhaps we can achieve a latch in a side-lying position. She
rolls all of a quarter of an inch. Since she said she breastfed
two others, I feel confident this will eventually work.

While checking the baby's mouth, Hope begins to make a
few meager sucking motions. Placing her against mom's side,
she licks milk, but makes no attempt to nurse. I return at 8 that
evening, and now only dad is in the room. As I change the baby's
diaper, I comment on the religious nature of their daughter's
name, and both parents nod in pleasure. Not knowing if they
have a religious affiliation, I make one simple comment.

"The Philippines is a diverse country, but they're strongly
Catholic, aren't they?"

"Yes, mostly Catholic."

Mom and I move on to attempt the feeding, and the baby
latches with some minor assistance.

"Would you mind coming over, Dad? I'd like you to see the
way I coax Hope to keep sucking. This'll be temporary. I think
she may need some coaxing for the first 24 hours." He jumps
to the bedside and mimics my actions, occasionally moving
the baby's arms. He watches as I place a blanket roll under
Hope's head to keep her aligned facing straight toward the
breast, since mom can't move well after the tubal. I let them
know who will see them the next day, but assure them I'll be
back the following morning and see them before discharge.

It's Thursday now, the day of discharge, and I read the baby's
chart before entering the room, and see that mom was giving

formula the day prior. I hadn't asked if she'd supplemented her other two or fed exclusively. This may have been her norm. It could have been due to her limited mobility after the tubal. I would soon find out. The baby is 48-hours-old.

They happily greet me as an old friend, and invite me to sit down.

"Did the baby wake up more, after I saw you Tuesday night?" I ask, admiring her little pink outfit spread out on the bed.

"Not much," dad tells me, "but then yesterday she feeding all day. We had to give her some formula because my wife, she didn't have enough milk. She say to me last night, "*Give me massage. Give me massage.*" She insisted. So I do. She remind me, in our country, this is what they do to bring more milk. I rub her back and rub her back, last night. And it work. Now she have lots of milk. We no need the formula."

They are grinning ear to ear. But it's only day 2 and I'm skeptical. Each day a little more milk comes, and the breasts usually *feel* heavier by 72 hours. Granted, mothers who've breastfed often have milk come in sooner, but still—Hope is barely 48-hours-old. I ask to see mom's breasts. And there they are—like firm melons. Another lesson in cultural breastfeeding practices.

Jamaicans: Two Encounters

*Culture is the blueprint for human behavior,
one that helps us to gain a clearer
understanding of individual behaviors. The
new mother is the product of all her history,
what she has learned about infants and infant
feeding and what she has seen.*

JAN RIORDAN

RN, PHD, IBCLC, LACTATION EDUCATOR

I read the chart before entering room 3357; 16-years-old, first baby, early and consistent prenatal care, marijuana positive on admission. The baby, according to the chart, has been nursing like a champ. I knock and am invited to enter. It's only mid-morning and there are two other women present. It looks like they've both spent the night—blankets and pillows strewn about, colorful clothing quite wrinkled. We greet and exchange congratulatory pleasantries.

Mama tells me about the birth. She'd gone natural, unusual for this region in general, certainly unusual for her young age. The grandma and great-grandma were ever present through the labor, coaching and encouraging. Their interactions are kind. They tell me they too breastfed their children for one to one-and-a-half years each. I provide basic teaching and offer to return when the baby is hungry, deciding to defer comment about marijuana until our next encounter.

In our region, it's standard practice to refer any mother admitted into Labor and Delivery who is street-drug positive, to Children's Protective Services (CPS), or 241-KIDS, as it's commonly called. Ohio is not Colorado, with liberal marijuana laws. Whether the mom is positive for heroin or weed, the referral process, handled by the social worker, is the same. Only for a short period in the late first decade of the 2000s, did CPS say they would not accept referrals for marijuana because the caseworkers were overloaded, and they had to prioritize. At some point, the caseload must have decreased because the social worker is busy making referrals again.

By the time I return in the afternoon, I read that the social worker has visited the mother. I re-enter the room and the energy has changed. Seen as an ally, they confide in me.

"We smoke daily and all our kids are healthy—smart, too."

They are Rastafari Jamaicans. I am curious and inquire as I sit on the edge of the bed while mama twirls her newborn's hair with her pinkie.

The elder women continue to explain that smoking is a daily ritual that opens their souls to peace. I read later that Rastafari's reject materialism and oppression of any kind, as well as sexual pleasure, but does this always apply? I don't ask. They are insulted by the inference that their daughter/granddaughter's ability to mother would be judged so harshly simply because she smokes weed daily. I listen sympathetically but gently acknowledge that cannabis is associated with double the risk of SIDS, and while there aren't many studies, some suggest that exposure in the first month is associated with lower motor skills at one year. They are unimpressed.

They will be going home today. The social worker stops me to say the family asked to speak with her again. They inform her that mama will be bottle-feeding, averting the issue of breastfeeding and marijuana. The social worker stares at me silently with a blank expression. I know what she's thinking and it's probably true. She'll go home and do what comes natural, which likely means following their culture's breastfeeding norm.

Some people feel the rain. Others just get wet.

BOB MARLEY

Like personalities, culture is multi-faceted. I see yet another example of this when I meet a 36-year-old Jamaican entrepreneur. My husband has told me to be on the lookout for the owner of *Mr. Green*, a cleaning service he frequently utilizes in his low-income housing field. He's told the owner to ask for me once she delivers. A couple weeks have passed and her name has already slipped my mind.

Today I am assigned room 3358 and enter to find a high cheek-boned mother cuddling her baby while filling out birth certificate forms. When she first speaks, it comes back to me immediately. You cannot mistake a Jamaican accent.

"May I ask, do you own a cleaning business?"

Now she seems to remember too. "You are Mr. Ron's wife? He has given me so much business. I like that man." We talk about the birth, the baby, and breastfeeding. She's nursed another child several years earlier. She is blasé about breastfeeding, seeming perplexed that Americans make such a big deal about it, as though it is a pure oddity that we obsess over pees and poops.

The consult is interrupted by a phone call. She apologizes and says she must take the call. I meander over to the computer and begin to chart, while she interrogates the person on the other end of the phone.

"What time did you get there? How many hours did it take? Did you speak to the landlord?" She hangs up and exhales a long breath. "I have to get back to work Monday," she declares.

"Oh, my goodness, the baby will only be 4-days-old, surely..." But she is already interrupting, "I'm the owner." It's really not my business, but I am catapulted into the problem-solving mode.

"Could you coordinate from home? Your milk will be in full force Monday, or...were you planning to take the baby with you?"

"No, no, not possible, I've got to do some of the cleaning. I just lost another employee. You have no idea how hard it is to find and keep good help in America. You'd never find this in my country."

I am intrigued, because, though I've never been there, I've wrongly assumed that Jamaicans are people who enjoy a lot of relaxing as they listen to their reggae music. I tell her as much and she laughs from her belly. "You Americans," she says, her voice trailing off. She tells me that Jamaicans, by and large, are industrious, hard workers who would never up and quit their job the way so many of her employees have. "We are raised to be the best at whatever we do."

I encourage her to ask some of her other employees to pick up the slack, but her demeanor tells me she has no confidence this plan will work. As bad as the U.S. maternity leave is, I can't think of a single situation where a mother would be expected to return to work *four days* after giving birth. But this is her work ethic and her business.

Far from the Congo, Her People, and Their Ways

Thinking that baby formula is as good as breast milk is believing that 30 years of technology is superior to three million years of nature's evolution.

CHRISTINA NORTHRUP

PHYSICIAN, AUTHOR

There are many Guatemalans and Hondurans that come to the U.S. fleeing from violence within their country. If they deliver here, we never discuss this history. The only questions I raise are where they gave birth to their other children and how they fed them. From another part of the world, Burundis too, fled the 1994 war with Rwanda. I've met many of them at the hospital and through a church affiliated with my parish.

But in 2015, the stories of refugees and refugee camps that have been dominating the news are primarily from Syria, Iraq, and Northern Africa. So it was surprising to meet a woman from deeper within the African continent, the Central Republic of the Congo, and inadvertently learn a bit of her story.

I'm embarrassed to say how little I know of what's happening in the African countries, and wonder if Europeans are better informed due to proximity or prior colonization. The U.S. is so isolated in comparison. To begin to counter this, my oldest daughter Jen and I take on the task of memorizing the names and locations of each country on the continent. From making up acronyms for the North, like MATLE (Morocco, Algeria, Tunisia, Libya, Egypt), I find ways to help me remember. Other countries are easier to recall due to a personal connection: Zimbabwe, where a friend taught on a Rhodes scholarship; Ghana, where my second daughter, Amy, planted trees in a rainforest. (I never fail to acknowledge to a Ghanaian that their country is the birthplace of Kofi Anan, a past secretary general of the United Nations. This always makes them smile.) Kenya, where a friend has been establishing schools for over ten years; Nigeria, home of a colleague with whom I authored a paper; Cameroon, home of my go-to tech guy from *Verizon*. We make our way north and south, then east and west on the map until we have it down pat.

On this particular day, I am told the mother in room 3120 has a question for me. Her language is unfamiliar, so I pick up the interpreter phone as I enter the room. I can access a Spanish interpreter in a matter of seconds, but this search takes 6 minutes before a gentleman comes on who speaks Wolof. As he introduces himself to she and I, she banters with him a bit, smile opening like daybreak across her face.

"What's her question for me?" I ask the interpreter.

"When can she start using formula?"

This is a frequent, and at times exasperating, conversation I have with many women, not just immigrants, but a non-American-born mother's situation is even more perplexing. I always begin by trying to understand her story, and today is no different.

"Do you have other children?" I ask him, while looking into her large dark eyes.

"Yes, seven, all here with her in the United States," the interpreter conveys.

"Did you breastfeed?" This makes her laugh and the interpreter joins in the chuckle.

"Of course!" she replies, sliding her hands to smooth the aqua hijab that covers her hair.

"How long did you breastfeed?"

She pauses while considering. "Different for each," she replies.

"Well, about how long?" I press.

"It's hard to recall because I was in a refugee camp many of those years." (*Many*? This gives me pause.)

It does not escape me that more than one child was born in a refugee camp as I listen to the interpreter rattling off the ages of the children. I would love to explore this part of her story, but now is not the time.

"I believe I gave them my breast for 2 or 2 1/2 years."

"And there you were, in a very difficult situation, doing something so good for the health of your babies." She smiles broadly, clearly proud of herself.

"Well, here in the U.S. it's equally good—the best!" I pause to let that settle in a few moments before continuing the conversation.

"Are you returning to work?" I ask this because it's a frequent reason to begin supplements, even when a mother hasn't secured a job.

"No, I just came to this country 8 months ago."

"So why would you want formula?"

"*Because it's available,*" she responds, with such an innocent expression on her face.

I tell her how not everything that's freely offered in the U.S. is worth the cost she'll pay in other ways. She's never suffered from a low supply, but if she begins to supplement, her body won't get the signals needed to understand how much to produce for this new offspring. I wait while the interpreter translates and she seems placated for now. When I ask if she's still willing to continue to only nurse her infant, she tucks her head slightly downward and speaks her native tongue into the phone.

"No worries," the interpreter tells me, "she understands what you are saying."

This scenario is indicative of a huge problem. I cannot help but heave an internal sigh. With her homeland having the 18th highest infant mortality rate in Africa, breastfeeding is saving lives. While outcomes in the U.S. are usually not as dramatic, it's nonetheless saving lives even here, and improving health for babies, as well as moms. But over her short 8-month stay in this country, formula has been promoted, albeit inadvertently, by our government's nutrition program, Women, Infant, and Children (WIC), and by the women who bottle-feed as they sit waiting in the clinic's corridors. We also know that WIC has singlehandedly been responsible for improving the rate of breastfeeding initiation for low-income mothers across the U.S. The story is never black and white. Yet, this mom, like so many, have come to think that formula is equivalent to their own milk and, worse, that it's simply part of assimilating to our culture. While in her own country, formula use would cause suspicion of a positive HIV status (and subsequent shunning), in the U.S., infant formula is too often looked at as the way of a wealthy New World, along with fries, sodas, and high-fructose corn syrup that will unwittingly begin to permeate her choices unless someone intervenes with culturally sensitive education. Her ticket to the U.S., along with her family, may have saved their lives. Now the task ahead is to save their health. Welcome to America.

Postscript

It's December 20th, and last night I slept with my 7-year-old granddaughter. When she quiets down, I ask Ava if she'd like to hear the story of her birth. This was a pre-Christmas tradition with my two girls, even into their 20s.

I recount my version of driving 10 hours to arrive, serendipitously, 6 hours before the birth. Ava's arrival had drama, obstacles, and a happy outcome. The story of this Congolese patient reminds me that women labor and deliver in foreign lands in, at times, hostile environments. I hope this mom will be able to recount her birth stories in ways that celebrate her trials and triumphs in the most adverse circumstances, and that she will come to see that offering her milk was a life-saving gift, and one of self-determination and personal power.

Karen and Other Latinas

*

The future is sending back good wishes, and
waiting with open arms.

KOBI YAMADA

I became friends with Concepcion and her family while they attended our small urban church. I've known them over 12 years. Her youngest daughter, Jennifer, tall and shy, was in eighth grade when she asked me to be her confirmation sponsor. Karen, 2 years older, is the more outgoing of the two. At 13 and 15, the girls seem so mature that it's easy to forget their young ages.

At Christmas Mass, Concepcion's eyes meet mine. They are sad and she seems preoccupied as we greet in the vestibule. She has just gotten her older son stabilized on medicine after some sort of a psychotic break. He had lost his college scholarship in the aftermath. When she hugs me she whispers, "Karen is pregnant." I feel for her. She must have had so many dreams for these children. I can see the once bright fabrics of hope for her children are fading, one by one. Concepcion tells me immediately who the dad is and it's clear she doesn't like him.

Karen is punished by not receiving any Christmas presents. I learn this after Christmas when I take her out to lunch. She tells me that she knows it may sound crazy, since she's only 15, but she and the boy really love each other and she sees her entire future with this young man. She counsels me not to worry, they'll be okay.

Karen has scheduled her first appointment in our hospital's OB office. I take her out 2 months later, along with Jennifer, and am happy to learn she's signed up for Centering classes, and that her boyfriend attends too. Centering prenatal care combines group education with private examinations. It's associated with a reduction in low birthweight babies, lengthening the spacing between pregnancies, nearly eliminating racial disparities associated with preterm birth, increased odds of breastfeeding at discharge from the hospital, and building confidence in the parents-to-be. The couple is driven to each appointment by her mother, who remains silent in the car. Karen vacillates between being frustrated with her mom, and being generous in understanding. She knows her mother's journey over 25 years ago from Honduras, and many of the years since, has not been easy, but it's hard to feel shunned by your mother.

We eat Italian that day, and the two sisters gorge on pasta, and gobble huge ice cream sundaes. Concepcion has now enrolled Jennifer in a youth modeling agency, and I can see that her mom is now channeling all her expectations on her last-born. When Karen is in the bathroom, I talk to Jennifer about how her mom's hopes are on her, the youngest child, and we talk about how that might feel. Jennifer knew this. She has a laid-back temperament and an internal drive of her own. I'm happy that, at least for now, Jennifer doesn't seem burdened with this pressure from her mom.

At our next outing, I meet Karen in the bleachers at her sister's volleyball tournament. Karen and I chat as we watch Jennifer, at ease on the court, lobbing balls over the net. Her mother and she are on speaking terms now. Karen is getting bigger and her due date is not far off. I have given her the simplest breastfeeding instructions, along with a crib and baby items. She is now 16 and genuinely confident.

The baby is born at our hospital, but even before my visit, Karen is having trouble with latch and has resorted to pumping. We attempt breastfeeding together using a nipple shield, but her newborn girl shows little interest. She'll be back in school in a few weeks and Karen reasons that pumping will be best. We talk about the pros and cons, and she makes limited attempts over the next few days at home where I visit to assist. Her supply is low, and even her pumping plans drift away.

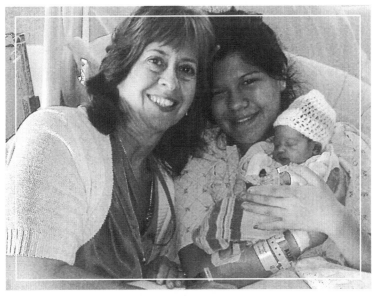

✳ *Chris, Karen, and Arianna.* ✳

I don't want Karen to let go of her plan to graduate high school and go to college, and so we talk about this the following month, days before she's to restart school, as I sit on her bed in the room she's always shared with Jennifer.

Jennifer quietly tells me she can put up with disturbed sleep because she just loves that little niece. It's the first time I've been upstairs, and the room is large and a disaster. Maybe this is how many teenagers live. I've forgotten what my girl's rooms looked like. Clothes are everywhere. Since Jennifer owns well over twice as many clothes as her sister, they're mostly hers. I chide them both to help me get the room picked up, and they cooperate in a way I think they wouldn't have if I'd been their mother.

The baby sleeps in Karen's bed, mattress on floor, while the new crib I'd gotten her, which can one day convert to a toddler bed, substitutes for a dresser, housing all the baby's clothes. Their mom works, providing elder care and doing some housekeeping on the side. She doesn't need to be picking up after two capable teen daughters, I surmise. After my visit, we go grocery shopping for diapers, and Karen tells me of her boyfriend troubles. He's skipping classes, and all he wants to do is play football. It takes another two years before she decides her feelings have changed and she cuts it off. Even so, she still involves him with their now toddler, encouraging him to be a fully participating dad.

Concepcion has a group of friends she gets together with every Saturday night. She sells raffle tickets, with proceeds going to her home country. The late nights aren't conducive to early-morning church anymore, but the girls surprise me one Sunday and show up at church after a long absence, toddler in tow. We go to the local *Big Boy* restaurant for brunch, and they update me about school, dating, home life, and the lanky toddler who's squirming in the booth. I admire them—committed, resourceful, happy teens. They function with limited resources. Their life has not been easy. But they still have goals that keep them fairly focused. While they may not have gotten the room-cleaning routine down, they are responsible in other ways. Karen is a conscientious mother, and Jennifer is a doting aunt. Concepcion revised her plans for the girls, loves them, and moved on, with new hopes and dreams for both of them. In fact, today, the girls attend the University of Cincinnati, and little Arianna begins kindergarten in the Fall of 2017.

* *

Hispanic mothers make up the majority of non-English speakers I've seen over the past 25 years. They typically hail from Guatemala, Honduras, or Mexico, but there are a few mothers from other Spanish-speaking countries as well. The few with a higher education are usually from South American countries and Spain.

In the late 90s, I sign up for a course offered by the hospital titled Medical Spanish. We practice by writing, then reading conversations we may have with a patient in our given field. Since then, I've completed most of my consults in Spanish. It's quite common to see a mom automatically roll to her side, if I comment that her baby is showing signs he's ready to nurse. There are so many Hispanic mothers who feed their babies lying on their side in bed that I don't think twice about it anymore. It seems to be part of their cultural norm.

Occasionally, if a mom has a native indigenous dialect, she listens to me attentively, and then turns to her husband with a quizzical look. He repeats what I've said in what sounds to me like the exact same words I've spoken, and she smiles at me knowingly. I can usually identify indigenous mothers because they often wear coats and hats, even in the warmest Cincinnati weather. They are the women who do not want cold food or drinks after a birth, believing this balance of hot-cold will help them heal sooner. If we don't feel we understand each other, I pick up the interpreter line on their bedside stand. This works fine for education, but if the speaker phone isn't working, and it's latch help that's needed, it's a bit comedic as we hold the phones in the crook of our necks to free our hands to position the baby. We both can't help but laugh as we struggle through.

If I've heard the phrase *no leche* once, I've heard it hundreds of times. I go through my spiel, explaining colostrum is the first milk, (*generalmente lo suficiente*- enough), discussing the baby's tiny stomach size, and then hand express drops so she can see. If she's a first-time mom, her worry is often assuaged, but I'm guessing that during the pregnancy, friends have solidified the idea of "no milk." If it is an experienced mom, she knows her breasts didn't "feel" full until she was home, and if she supplemented early after other births, it's not easy now to convince her that her milk is sufficient. Even if she continues to exclusively breastfeed, she is often skeptical. Sometimes, on subsequent mornings, I learn that she has asked someone else for formula and they've obliged. That day's conversation then involves damage control—how to go from *los dos*, both, to solely breastfeeding as soon as her breasts become heavy. The self-fulfilling prophecy of not having enough milk is realized if she continues to supplement once her milk is fully in, because the baby isn't nursing often enough to build an adequate supply, in the delicate supply-demand balance. Yet there are other times when a mother understands my explanation of the immunologic properties of her early milk, and that the doctors want the baby to have all of these benefits, and she seems calmed and fascinated with my explanation of the best way to make lots of milk, and I happily find she's exclusively breastfed her entire hospital stay.

Well before our hospital was certified as Baby-Friendly, the manager of the Mother-Baby unit asked me to track our exclusive breastfeeding rate, qualifying that I should skip the Hispanics because they "always" supplement. I decided to track both, and found that Hispanics supplemented slightly less than non-Hispanics. I presented this data to the staff with the manager present. If you approach the mother with this false assumption, you inadvertently undermine exclusive breastfeeding. The repetition can be exhausting, explaining the benefits of exclusive breastfeeding, and the risks of early supplementation, to a mother whose goal already is to breastfeed. But I have infinite patience with the mothers. I have little patience when the system undermines breastfeeding, often inadvertently sabotaging her goal by not establishing policies and protocols that protect this fragile bond. It's not wrong to give the mother formula at her request. It's wrong not to educate her about the implications of early supplementation, and then blame her for not being committed.

* * *

You say gently to yourself: This person has
feelings, emotions, and thoughts—just like me.
This person, at some point in his or her life,
has been sad, disappointed, hurt, or confused—
just like me. This person has, in his or her life,
experienced physical and emotional pain and
suffering—just like me.

CHADE-MENGE TAN
SEARCH INSIDE YOURSELF

I'm helping a quiet 17-year-old mom, whose day-old son is breastfeeding with ease. She'd been seen yesterday by the lactation consultant whose first language is Spanish. The mom's 18-year old boyfriend sits on the couch, playing on his phone. While I'd begun the conversation in Spanish, I ask if they speak English, as often the teens do. She is silent, while he holds his fingers an inch apart and says, "A little," as the smile on his face reveals a dimple on his right cheek.

"Are you in school," I query? Both nod yes. "Same school?"

"Yes."

"I suppose, math may be easiest to learn if your teachers only speak English."

"It's hard," he answers, and his lip goes up on one side, in an acknowledgment that he knows I understand their difficulty.

"How long have you been in the country?" I ask.

He is only speaking for himself now, and replies, "Since I was 4. My sister and I came from Guatemala."

"With your parents?"

"No, it was just us," he says, still smiling.

"Well, how old was *she*?" I am thinking she must have been old enough to be his mom, and am astounded at his answer.

"14."

"14? I repeat in disbelief. "Just the two of you?"

"Ya." He has to see the look of astonishment on my face, and he seems to hold himself a little higher in his seat on the couch, as if to indicate some pride that they survived the trek.

"Wow," is all I can say back.

How I would have loved to hear his story, if he remembered, at that tender age, what their journey entailed, but we had a brief encounter and I would not be meeting them again, and there was breastfeeding basics to review, as their baby fed contentedly in long sucking bursts. I asked which language she preferred I use.

"Spanish," she replied, with no hesitation. We finished the consult in her native language.

I brought dad over to the mother's bedside, and we talk about how he can help her as she breastfeeds, positioning pillows, getting her something to drink, holding the baby skin-to-skin, rocking his son. They were discharged that afternoon having exclusively breastfed during the hospital stay.

Postscript

I began this story with a quote about a mindfulness exercise, meant to help me give focused, compassionate care, and listening to my patients and their families. I don't in any way want to judge or minimize the profound differences in our life experiences. Yet, we share a common humanity that not only binds us together, but I hope reminds us that we're on this life-boat together, that we're here to help each other. What these patients and families offer me is as valuable as what I offer them.

＊ ＊ ＊ ＊

The young mother from the Dominican Republic is surrounded by family: daddy, grandma, great-grandma, and niece. They are chatting happily in Spanish among themselves as I enter the room. Mommy had an emergent C-section only 21 hours ago, but she is moving about well today. I tell her that just from reading her chart when I came in today, I think her baby girl is the best breastfeeder on the unit. Everyone smiles in satisfaction.

"Did you happen to breastfeed your daughter?" I ask the grandma.

"Oh, yes, we are a breastfeeding family. But I didn't do it long with her. My father died when she was 9 days old, and I think the stress decreased my supply. I only lasted 6 weeks. But others, I nursed longer. My father was one of 12 children, and my uncle, the youngest of the family, tells me he remembers breastfeeding until he was 7!"

"Ah, the world-wide weaning age is 4.2 years, so somebody has to be nursing as long as your uncle for that to average out. What country are you all from?" I query.

"The Dominican Republic," they all chime in together. "Except my daughter was born here in the U.S.," the grandma informs me.

The mother wants to be taught the football hold, and she moves to a chair as I change the baby's diaper. As I undress the baby, I say a few words in Spanish to grandma, and she is off and running in her native tongue. I can keep up, but I tell her that it's easiest for me when the topic is breastfeeding. This makes her laugh, and we continue speaking in her native tongue until the mother is ready to receive her newborn. Showing her how to hand express her milk, we all see that it drips a golden yellow. While the great grandma "ah's," I explain to the dad how valuable this first milk is to his baby's health. He nods in understanding, and then reluctantly tells the mama good-bye. When he leaves, the grandma says that she's sent him home to sleep, and though he doesn't want to, she thinks it's best he be rested before the baby comes home.

"I can only stay a month," she says, as she folds the baby's sleeper. The older women listen as I give the mom basic instructions. There'll be time for details tomorrow, since she'll be staying three or four days. There is a confidence in the air that's palpable. Their understanding is breastfeeding "just works."

As we discuss nutrition briefly, grandma brings me a glass bottle that looks to hold about 16 ounces. The contents are tan in color, and there seems to be flecks of something floating around in it. The color and texture don't seem right, but I ask if it's Atole, the corn-based drink that many mothers from Mexico and Central America drink to increase their supply.

"It's oatmeal, milk, water, vanilla extract, and a little sugar. Our culture finds it to help a mom's milk supply and after my troubles, I want her to get off to a good start. Oatmeal is okay, right?"

I assure her it's great, and she gives me a warm hug and thanks me for coming to help her daughter. I move on to the Peruvian in the room next door.

The Italians

I have done what is mine to do.

FRANCIS OF ASSISI

It's early spring 2000, and I'm assigned to a lovely doctor-doctor couple from Italy. They're eager and receptive to learn all they can about breastfeeding in the 45 minutes I spend with them during their two-day hospital stay. They're here for their residency program, and are assuming they'll be returning to Italy.

On day 2, when Gabriella finishes breastfeeding the baby, I tell them I am leaving in less than a month for Europe. It's our first trip across the water, and we're celebrating our 25th wedding anniversary. We've chosen this specific tour because it's the only one that has a stop in Assisi, birthplace of Saint Francis. The couple is Catholic, and they are thrilled to tell me that they both grew up near Assisi, in a small town in the Umbrian region of Central Italy. They understand why a stop in Assisi is a priority, and assure me that we will fall in love with the medieval town. Besides this, I tell them excitedly, we will be meeting up with Father John Quigley, the Franciscan who braved the 23 inches of snow that had fallen the night before our wedding to arrive in Akron, Ohio to perform the ceremony. Though residing in Geneva now, he's conducting a pilgrimage in Assisi on the very day we'll be there. Our plans intrigue them, and they are in awe of the serendipitous meet-up. They share travel tips about their homeland, and tell me a few essential words and phrases I should know in Italian, wishing me *buona fortuna*, as I depart their room.

Not long after our trip, Gabriella calls with questions about pumping and milk storage guidelines that she'll need to know before returning to her residency program. I ask about Teresa Clare, and she swoons on about the love of her life. She then asks about the trip, which I think is the real reason for her call. I describe the couple we met, a husband-wife psychiatric nurse team, originally from the island of Mauritius, off the coast of Madagascar, but who now reside in England. She listens attentively as I explain that all hospital staff were recently assigned to watch a video about cultural diversity, and that it was all about the three distinct cultures who live in harmony on this tiny island of Mauritius.

While in Assisi, we stop at San Damiano, a 13th-century chapel. I tell her that afterward, we dug a small hole in the dirt of the hillside outside the chapel, planting a lock of hair from each of our four children, praying that they will be guided in their career choices. The boys are still in high school, the girls, in college. My Italian patient understands the symbolism. At the end of his life, Francis is quoted as saying, "I have done what is mine to do. May Christ teach you what is yours." Gabriella's sigh expresses understanding, and she tells me that she can't wait to tell her husband our story when he's finished with hospital rounds today.

We have been fortunate. Our own career paths, (my lactation consulting and Ron's in low-income housing development) have been clear to us. They are our mission and passion. I can only hope that others are given the opportunity to fulfill theirs, our children included.

Indian Interfaces

*Have a big enough heart to
love unconditionally, and a broad
enough mind to embrace the differences
that make each of us unique.*

DB HARROP

A small, framed picture of a middle-aged woman wearing traditional Indian garb sits prominently on her bedside stand as I enter the room. Like the woman in the picture, Neela wears a red dot, known as a Bindi, in the lower middle of her forehead. I comment that it's lovely and inquire as to its meaning. She tells me that the meaning varies.

"Yes, it can be simply decorative, but it's also spiritually symbolic of inner guidance. It is usually worn by married women, but men can wear it too." I learn that it also hearkens to unity, when creation first began. I find this last fact especially fascinating, given I am being told this by a young woman who has just given birth 9 hours ago.

As her baby nurses after some latch assistance from me, Neela's eyes light up in understanding, "So this is a good feeding, I can tell. She's hardly stopping." She listens attentively as I explain how milk is made. Her mother, who will be arriving from India in two weeks, has already assured her, well before birth, that there is nothing to worry about; so she has an air of calm and confidence about breastfeeding, unusual for a first-generation immigrant here, with no family other than her husband. She is pleased when she says her mother will be staying for 6 months. What a gift of support, I think.

The nurse arrives, a single middle-aged woman, herself from India. Her nurse asks, even with me present, if the mother thinks her baby is getting enough milk. For many first-time breastfeeders, this question alone can be like the corrosive acid that sits atop an old battery rendering it inert. "Are you sure?" She continues to press while I interject noting some obvious signs of effective feeding. I make a mental note to speak privately to the nurse. I consider her questioning a projection of her own lack of confidence. Colostrum, the first milk, is generally quite enough. Despite the nurse's intimidating questions, Neela responds confidently that she has no doubt. As she says this, she tips her fingers with reverent serenity toward the picture on the bedside stand, saying a name unrecognizable to me, "She will guide me."

I can almost see the hair on the nurse's back rise. She begins to scurry about the room, straightening the patient's belongings; she's known to be a good housekeeper. I'm jotting notes in my chart as she does the room sweep, but I look up when she begins telling the mother she should learn about Jesus, her Lord, and Savior. I am Christian myself, but I see this as way out of line in a patient-nurse relationship, where the inherent power resides with the professional. "You should really look into the Bible. You'd be surprised," she claims. The mother offers a kind reply, unperturbed.

It is then that I make the connection that the pretty lady in the picture is some type of spiritual leader, and not her mother. I wait until the nurse leaves and ask. She tells me Hinduism is practiced by the majority in her homeland, that it was the faith of Mahatma Gandhi. Later, I read he described it as "the relentless pursuit of truth through non-violent means." The woman in the picture is her renowned yogi master and teacher.

The mother was about to tell me where she practiced yoga when her bubbly perinatologist, Dr. Vinita, enters the room. In a heavy Indian accent, she speaks, "*Vhat? Vhat?* Are you talking about meditation? Chris, we should go together. It's on Friday nights; very healthy for the mind and body." After this, she proceeds to tell the mother she'd had trouble with her supply with her first baby, born in India. "I *vas* a nervous wreck. So much worry, did not help." But then, she continues, she had her second at our hospital and I helped get them off to a good start, and she had no trouble with supply that time. She also concedes that her aunt shipped her fenugreek from India, an herb touted to increase a milk supply. She swears it did the trick. Enthusiastically, the doctor tells the mother and me that in India, it is even fed to cows after they give birth to assure a robust supply of milk. And this makes the doctor chuckle aloud. She is off on a mini-lecture about health practices in India, telling us that Reglan, a prescription drug sold in the U.S. for stomach problems, is often passed out after deliveries "like communion wafers" to build mothers' milk supply. An unexpected side-effect is that it raises levels of the milk hormone, prolactin.

I mention something an Indian intern said to me during the previous month's lactation lecture. His mother had a low supply, and fed him solely at night, allowing her two lactating sisters, his aunts, to nurse him by day. They both nod, as if this made perfect sense to them. I marvel at the many practices different from my own in lactation, culture, and religion. As the petite perinatologist strides toward the door, she stops again, the top of her head inches from my nose. "Call me Chris. Let's go meditate." Though Dr. Vinita was unavailable, I went to the patient's yoga center near the hospital the following Friday just that once.

Postscript

Lillias Folan was a Cincinnati-based yoga practitioner who hosted a PBS television show. I occasionally watched a bit, but only because it dovetailed with Sesame Street. She closed her program consistently with the word, Namaste. "The god in me, greets the god in you." I never learned its meaning until years later, when I cared for many Indian patients. It is a beautiful way to greet anyone.

Smeared Dates on an Egyptian Babe

Before I knock and announce myself,
I look at the name. It's foreign,
seems Arabic, with its y-a-h ending.
She might speak English, or French
if she were from some northwest
African country—or just speak Arabic.
I'll soon find out.

Muslim mothers respond warmly when I
greet them with their traditional
As-*salamu alaykum*, or say,
In sha allah—God willing,
as I let them know to expect
their milk to arrive in abundance
on day of life three.

Upon entering the room, I see her
Muslim garb, learn she is Egyptian,
non-English speaking. But before I can
pick up the interpreter phone, a portly
bearded man, addresses me in
English, inviting me to be seated
near the mother's bed.

I ask if the five-year-old girl in the room
is their daughter. *No, no, hers*, he points.
I'm the uncle. This leads me to think
she has breastfeeding experience.
– and she nods her head, seeming to understand

at least some. I visit in English,
then use an interpreter for education.

Advancing to the crib, I see a chubby baby
bundled in white with some odd black sticky
substance smeared around her rosebud lips.

If not for the scent, it could have been
meconium, that initial tarry stool that
newborns poop out in the early days of life.
I'm left wondering –If not meconium, then what?

What is this, I ask, and he frantically
begins an explanation that meanders its
way around my concern. I see the mother's
eyes. Without understanding the words, she
hears my tone and knows I am alarmed.
Solid food isn't recommended before
six months of age.

I knew a pediatric resident who disregarded this
guide and poured rice cereal into his own
2-month-old's nighttime bottle, in the
hope of a better night's sleep. But this
is no 2-month-old and he is no pediatrician.
And so the question sits between us like
an interpreter waiting to translate.

He points to the older daughter,
saying she's evil, spits hateful things,
her tongue, a weapon. The girl, despite a
language barrier, seems to know he is talking about her.
He says he is protecting the second-born daughter

from the same fate by this ritual of smearing
her mouth with dates.

The uncle assures me he has chewed these
dates into a pulp and fed her nothing.
I must look incredulous standing there—
American, foreigner in the room.
The daughter begins to shriek –
expletives sounds in Arabic, he looks aghast,
saying, *See, see, she's evil.*

In America, we might say she is
a strong-willed child, we might be resolute
in curbing her behavior, we might laugh
it off and suggest everyone else relax,
she's a child after all. But I am the guest
in this 8x8 hospital-room-home and I am
there to assure her baby receives only mother's milk.

Postscript

There are over one hundred varieties of dates grown in many North African, European,
and Middle Eastern countries. This is one example of power ascribed to a food from
another culture to which most Americans, me included, may be oblivious. Respecting
the culture of our patients affords us the opportunity to learn from and about them.

Liberated Libyan Physicians

*I would like it to be thought that I had listened
carefully to what patients and others have
told me, that I've tried to imagine what it was
like for them, and that I tried to convey this.
And to use a Biblical term, bore witness.*

OLIVER SACKS

NEUROLOGIST, AUTHOR

I learned a little about the North African country of Libya when a husband-wife physician team was under my care. Many foreign-born patients express gratitude when I show interest, and at least some rudimentary knowledge of their homeland. And so it was with this family. Breastfeeding was proceeding as expected, and when the teaching was complete, I asked how long they'd been in the U.S. I learn they'd had quite an adventure arriving in Cincinnati for their residency program two years earlier.

A year before the 2012 attack on the U.S. embassy in Benghazi, the U.N. had unanimously voted to enforce a No-Fly Zone over Libya. This was a consequence of attacks on civilians by the Libyan government itself. It lasted six months, ending after the capture and death of the country's former leader, Muammer Gaddafi. It was in the middle of this very six-month period that the couple had planned a flight to the U.S. to begin their residency program.

They were thrust into their own crisis, packing their belongings and traveling by ship, 400 miles to Turkey's shore. Unlike the more recent refugees arriving in Turkey in 2016 who are fleeing poverty, war, and oppression, these immigrants did not have to pay bribes, travel in a rickety boat, or worry that they would be lost at sea. They did, however, have to hide the fact that the West was their final destination. Upon arriving in the U.S., they were welcomed into our country and the local medical community, where they began their training in July 2011.

Passing the baby over to dad, I slid the baby down dad's scrubs, easily nesting him skin-to-skin. Dad reclined the chair and patted his newborn. The three of us continued to talk about their homeland and its notorious leader. I was fascinated, listening to this insider perspective. I knew little of Gaddafi. I was aware he was fashion-conscious and rather unpredictable. "Most Americans would never believe it, but he wasn't *all* bad," she assured me, as her dark brown eyes, focused on my own. He'd taken over in 1969, and in the early years, he was credited with raising Libya's income to the fifth highest in Africa, and with improving education. Yet he was an enigma. On one hand, he was a strong supporter of Nelson Mandela. On the other hand, he was loyal to Uganda's brutal dictator, Idi Amin. He had immense personal wealth due to the extraction of oil in the country. Some estimated he was worth 90 *billion* dollars.

He had unusual interests. The couple explained that his money financed many anti-nuclear movements. What surprised me most was when this mother said that Gaddafi used his personal wealth to secure the release of hostages in more than one country. The most publicized exchange was his personal $25 million dollars he'd handed over to Filipino terrorists for the successful release of six Westerners. Westerners, mind you.

Here in room 3366, I saw two new immigrants who'd just birthed an American citizen, and I was given a good lesson in both history and human character I would never have gotten from a history book. I saw resilience in their eyes, as they spoke passionately about the homeland they love. Certainly, poverty did not hold them back. They did not have to risk their lives in ways we've seen in 2016, when poor citizens of northern Africa, fleeing violence, board unsafe vessels to immigrate to Mediterranean countries. I will never forget the heart-wrenching image of the bodies of three children washed ashore in Turkey, amidst this crisis. No, this family will more than survive, in part, because these parents had financial means after receiving a good public education, via an academic system that improved during the reign of their notorious leader.

The Girl from the Land of Mount Everest

Remember me as the one who woke up.

BUDDHA

Her features remind me of the Sherpas: ovoid eyes, bronze, leathery skin. When I ask about her hometown, I learn Nepalese don't talk of towns; they only say they are from the east or west, or south or north. The direction that matters to them is upward. She tells me a bit of her story as I watch her change the baby's diaper with the awkwardness of a first-time mom. She lived at 9,000 feet elevation, surrounded by mountains. Mountains everywhere you look, she said. They seem to have left an indelible mark on her, one that is both physical and mental.

When they coaxed you to deep breathe in labor, did you surprise your nurse at how well you did this? She nods. It's an accurate guess because her lung capacity is so much greater from the thin air she breathed for 13 years. Despite the passing of time, memories of Everest, its 29,000 feet, have not faded in the least.

Now, at 21, she's given birth to her firstborn, a black-haired daughter, more fair-skinned than mom. She seems timid, listening attentively to basic guidance about how to breastfeed. Her mother-in-law sleeps on the couch. Blankets are over her body and head, reddish winter hat sticking out amidst the covers in the middle of May. She tells me that her sister-in-law has an older baby, and she told this mama that offering her milk plus formula is best, fattening the baby up quickly. As I sit next to her, I let her know how common this misperception is. People around the world seem to love fat babies. Yet this extra fattening isn't healthy for babies. They can grow up to be chubby toddlers, then plump teens. *Your daughter should grow well on your milk alone.*

She tells me that in Nepal no one is ever sick. She was so young when she left; I doubt she was really aware of diseases in her country. But I know that GI illnesses from contaminated water sources, leprosy, TB, even HIV, exist there. But maybe in her town, she never knew of an ill relative or friend. She says she is amazed at how many Nepalese in America have "this disease or that." When she hears that anything other than her milk increases her baby's risk for illness, she is quick to remind me that this is her first baby, and she wants to learn everything she can.

A friend has told her to give the baby water. *Another common misperception,* I assure her. The largest component of milk (and formula, for that matter) is water. "Babies need water, but from nowhere else than your milk—even if you'd delivered in the hottest month of our summer season." She listens attentively.

She asks about the baby sleeping in bed with her. "How does that work?" she wondered aloud. I want her to understand that proximity matters, that in the first year, it's safest if she stays near mom in the bassinette. *Don't put your baby in a far-off room where you won't hear each other,* I caution.

Before we part, I am called down the hall to see a 26-year-old mother who is asking for a bottle. They tell me she's from a refugee camp in Nepal. A climber who reached the summit was asked why he conquered Everest. "Because it's there," was his reply. I am hoping that both of these moms see that what is *there* is milk and that they can succeed in their hopes to breastfeed. I walk down the hall and begin the conversation anew.

The Thriving Ethiopian Child and the Bike She Covets

*Knowing that we can be loved exactly as
we are gives us all the best opportunity for
growing into the healthiest of people.*

FRED ROGERS

I enter room 3357 late in the day, after realizing the mom had birthed after the 8am census had been printed. It's now after *quiet-time*, which all mothers are provided so they have a chance to nap or hold their babies skin-to-skin with no staff interruption. My knock awakens both parents and I apologize, saying I am leaving in an hour, and want to make sure mom is seen. She shakes her head and shrugs her shoulders as if to say, "not a problem."

Her daughter is stirring as I ask about how breastfeeding has gone so far.

"She's fed twice, already." But dad interrupts and corrects her.

"Three times. You fed her in the other room." She nods in agreement as he points in the direction of labor and delivery.

They are thin, with light brown skin, and speak English with only a slight accent. I'm glad because Amharic interpreters are hard to come by. I make an educated guess as to their origins. There are clues. With her high cheek bones and skin smooth as silk, she's stunning, even at 40. There are also two pots of food on the bedside table. I never know what's inside, but the smell and her looks are distinctly Ethiopian. They show me one pot, and dad says it's wheat rice and sorghum, and a type of special butter. There's a scent of turmeric in the room too, and he tells me that the other pot had porridge in it. "You know what I mean, porridge?" he asks. "It's like a stew."

"Of course, a stew. Are you Ethiopian?" I ask, as I change the baby's diaper and glance at my notes. I read it's baby number five.

"You remember us!" the father, who looks about 50, says with a pleased smile. But I don't remember. However, this prompts me to ask about the prior births.

"All the rest were in Africa," mom says, "with the exception of the last. You helped us while she was in the Intensive Care— and loaned us a pump, too."

"Aw, how long did you breastfeed?" I inquire. "And when was this?"

"Well we tried to breastfeed, but she was so tiny. She was a little more than 23 weeks at birth."

I drop my jaw, and this inserts a pause, and we each know, silently, that their child is a miracle. "It was even hard to feed her by bottle. Do you want to see a picture?" she asks, while simultaneously latching the baby I've handed her and thumbing through pictures on her phone. She begins to laugh as she's browsing, and I sit down where she's patted the edge of the bed.

"This is a video of her in *Toys R Us*. She's begging for a bike."

I watch, seeing only Aynalem with rows of bikes in the backdrop. She's darling, in her pink matching shorts and top. She may be begging, but she's quite shy about it. I ask, "Is she 4? 5?"

"She's just about to turn 6 in this picture." We listen to the audio, and I hear Mom repeatedly saying, "Ask your daddy, go on, ask your daddy." Apparently, she's going to show the video to her husband later. I'm amazed at how Americanized they seem.

"In this picture, it's only been two weeks since her trach was removed. She's still got her G-tube."

"I'd never guess," I say. "She looks great!"

With this new piece of information though, I realize the journey of the past 5 years of their family life has likely been dictated by the needs of Anyalem. Dozens and dozens of monthly appointments with all the specialists needed for her care to become the little girl I see in the video. I wonder if she eats anything at all by mouth, or even a little; but I don't ask about the G-tube where likely most of her nutrition of liquid and pureed foods are passed into the stomach. They beam as we re-watch the video together, just like I watch and re-watch my own grandkids' clips.

"Well," I ask, waiting for the punch line, "did she get the bike?"

"Not that day. We surprised her on her birthday," Mom says, as her baby continues to nurse away.

I smile, and as I look up at Dad, inquire, "And what's this baby's name?"

"Opinion."

He must see that I look a bit perplexed and interjects, "Oh, her name? I thought you meant mine. Mine means *opinion*. Her name is Simbo. S-i-m-b-o. It means, hm, *colorful* or like *natural attractiveness*."

"Sweet. And her big sister's?"

"Her name means *light of the world*," Daddy says with pride written all over his expression.

Collateral Damage in Eastern Europe

*What do you pack to pursue a dream, and
what do you leave behind?*

SANDRA SHARPE

How did peace efforts connect this lactation consultant with a breastfeeding researcher in Sweden and a Serbian physician? In November 2015, someone in my writing workshop wrote a piece to commemorate the 20th anniversary of the Dayton Peace Accord. This was a peace agreement between the Serbian government and the fledgling governments of Bosnia and Croatia. Like this fellow writer, I was at the Dayton Air Force Base, outside the fence in 1995, praying for peace and a successful Accord for countries at war 5,000 miles away.

In 1994, a few of us in our faith community spearheaded a prayer campaign by developing a table-tent prayer card, highlighting the crisis, the victims, and the leaders that needed prayer. Two thousand prayer cards were sent around the world, due to our connection with an NGO in Geneva: Franciscan International.

One morning, months later, I received a personal note of gratitude from a woman who was part of the secular Franciscans in Sweden. I recognized her name because Dr. Kerstin Nyqvist has published research on ways NICU staff can intervene to support breastfeeding very low birthweight infants. It's a small world.

Shortly after the Accord, I took care of a first-time mother–physician originally from Serbia. Once the task of breastfeeding education was complete, we talked about her country and the recent war. In most circles, the leader of the Serbs, Slobodan Milosevic, was considered the culprit in inciting the ethnic cleansing that went on for several years. The intolerance from people of different religions was at the heart of the genocide. I'd honestly never thought about the impact of the war on the Serbian people in the former Republic of Yugoslavia. This was, in part, a consequence of slipping into dividing the world into two narrow categories of good and evil. It just didn't allow me to see the suffering of both sides.

As the baby quietly nursed, Ana spoke passionately about the pain her people endured. Indeed, her family lost everything valuable when it was seized by the state, including banked money, jewelry, homes, and heirlooms. Everything went to fuel the war machine. Everyone lived in fear. She shook her head, still in disbelief that this fate had descended upon her family, so removed and innocent of war-like intentions. As her voice trailed, I heard in it the residual concern for all the family members she'd left behind. Leaving her country did not mean she'd abandoned the pain. Our conversation was a startling reminder that all sides had loss of life and life as they knew it. And yet, she was fortunate enough to find her way to the U.S., reinvent her life, and pass it on to the next generation.

Three Generations of Senegalese

*A nation's culture resides in the
hearts and in the soul of its people.*

MAHATMA GANDHI

Browsing her chart, I see she's only breastfed once and supplemented with formula nine times in the baby's first 24 hours of life. It would be easy to justify placing her low on the priority list, but something makes me take a second look. It was a delivery very similar to my own firstborn: not descending, forceps used, mother's bottom swollen, needing a catheter until the swelling subsides enough that she pees on her own.

I knock and am invited to enter. The nurse is there changing the baby's diaper, and though she'd fed nearly an ounce of formula an hour prior, being handled has made Awa begin to fuss. I ask if we can attempt a feeding with mother in the semi-reclined position we call "laid back." Her obstetrician, Amy, enters. She is enthused about breastfeeding, and tells the mother she'd like to stay and watch the strategies I use to help the baby attach. This first-time mother agrees without fanfare, but we are unsuccessful, in part because the baby is probably still full, and in part because her nipples retract when she begins to hold her breast, making it likely that the baby will slide off. There are ways around this, and I give Assiante my cell number to call me when the baby is showing signs of hunger. In the meantime, I review eight basic points about breastfeeding. The grandmother, now awake on the couch, is listening, though I don't know if she speaks English. I ask the mother where she's from. Senegal. "Ah, parlez-vous francais?" I know the answer before I ask, since Senegal was a French colony. She has been here a few years. I asked her mother how long she breastfed the patient. In French, she replies, "Two years." with a smile beaming now. "*Tres bien*," I say with affirmation.

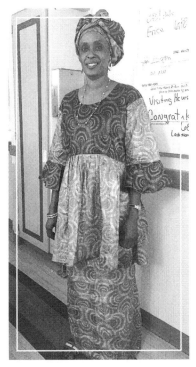

✳ *Senegalese Family Support.* ✳

When I return late morning, Assiante is determined to get Awa latched. She succeeds with the use of a shield over the nipple, making sustained sucking workable. She tells me that when she latched after the birth, it was merely a few sucks. I assure her that she will eventually be able to latch without the shield, but for now, she is content to just watch her newborn nurse. I return again late afternoon, and now the room is full of company. A man, a woman, and, I learn, the woman's 14- and 10-year-old daughters. When I say I am going to help Mom breastfeed, and then have Grandma offer a half-ounce using a cup, the woman steps up assertively and says she will do the supplementing. The baby is nursing even better than in the morning and, as we watch, the mother tells me that these are her nieces and their mother–

her sister. Her sister smiles toward me as she speaks a native dialect with her own mother.

"I told my mother that you helped me breastfeed both my girls," her sister says, smiling broadly.

"Ah, that just shows you how much I'm aging. How long did you breastfeed?

"Eleven months, but then only six months for the younger girl who went on strike about that time."

I ask the girls where they go to school.

"Walnut Hills High School and Dater Montessori."

I ask the older daughter if she is learning Latin.

"Yes."

"Of course—you're bright!" But she tucks her chin demurely, and says that Latin and French are very similar.

"So, you speak four languages then?" Now everyone is smiling, obviously proud of this young lady.

Next, I ask her mother if she spoke English 14 years ago when I first helped her.

"Oh, yes. I learned English in college."

College? I realized I had made an inaccurate assumption that an African immigrant would not have been to college in her own country.

A man, all smiles, enters the room. The patient seems so pleased to see him, and comfortable nursing as he enters, that I ask if it's her husband.

"No, it's my brother. He was the first one to help me try to get Awa to latch yesterday after the birth."

"Ah, he's a dad?"

"No, he just knew that was what should happen after the birth. Come see," she says. "Awa's feeding."

He meanders to her side and smiles. "Good girl, Awa."

Now that's a breastfeeding-friendly culture.

The Moroccans Who Forgot Their French But Remember Their Daily Rituals

There are a hundred different ways to kneel and kiss the ground.

RUMI

I knock, and the father invites me in. His wife is freshening up in the bathroom. He speaks English with ease and we chat as we await his wife. Now and again, he reaches into the pram and pats his newborn reassuringly. The room faces the front of the hospital, and from the large picture window, I see the Ohio and American flags flapping in the wind, a great gesture of welcome. The medivac helicopter's blades spin above as it prepares to land on the hospital's roof. Someone unknown to the dad and mom is being air-cared into our Trauma Unit, potentially on the opposite end of the birth-death cycle than this joyful father and child before me.

His wife comes and sits down on the couch next to him, and I introduce myself. She's smiling with her deep brown eyes, and her hair pulled back in a bun. I ask where they are from, and he tells me Morocco.

"Ah," I begin, "*Je suis consultante de l'allaitement maternel.*" They both look sheepishly at me, half recognizing my greeting. Dad tells me they've both forgotten their French. "We haven't spoken it in so long, only in school, really."

This surprises me, and I tell them that my twin nieces, Theresa and Emily, took French six years in middle and high school, and their final class trip was to Morocco. In turn, the dad tells me that Moroccans may also speak Arabic, English, and Spanish.

"In fact, Spain and Morocco once considered building a bridge across the Strait of Gibraltar, to connect us," he explains, with an air of national pride. "It's only about 600 kilometers away." I am doing my mental math and figure that to be about 1,000 miles.

"Now that would have been one long bridge," I reply.

I turn to the mother who seems to understand only some of what I say, as her eyes go to her husband for translation, and they speak in whispered Arabic. Per protocol, we don't ask family to interpret, so Mom and I move over to the bed, and I reach for the interpreter phone on the nightstand. I dial the 800 number, enter the code, ask for a female, and an Arabic interpreter introduces herself within minutes. We begin by talking about her sore nipples, and are deep in conversation when from the corner of my eye, I see Dad clicking away on his phone, replacing it in his pocket as he rolls out a prayer rug. He must have been on an app telling him where Mecca is so he knows how to position himself on the floor. He prays and we talk. She latches the baby with only a brief wince and then a smile.

"Much better," the interpreter tells me, and we continue our conversation. She understands to keep a diary of feedings, and wets and poops to show the pediatrician at the first appointment scheduled two days after discharge. She nods in understanding as the interpreter repeats that her son will show her signs of hunger and breastfeed eight to twelve times each 24-hour day. She asks questions, and Daddy prays on.

A friend recently emailed while touring Dubai. Carol, his wife, is the former long-time travel editor for the *Seattle Times*. She is writing a story about Middle-Eastern cuisine in Dubai. Tom's letter informs me that all hotel rooms in Dubai have an arrow on the ceiling so that Muslim occupants always know which way to bow in prayer toward Mecca.

I pause to take in the scene before me, looking at the three of them in this small hospital room and know what I see will be their daily ritual; he, praying 5 times each day, she, nursing, 8 to 12.

Chapter Three

THE LANGUAGE INTERPRETERS

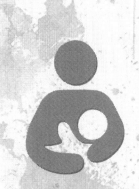

Language Interpreters

I am an interpreter of stories.

NAT KING COLE

Our hospital has had the best fortune when hiring language and sign interpreters. Every one of them is so professional, personable, and willing to go above and beyond in assisting our patients. The interpreters who were born in other countries attest to having been breastfed and those with children breastfed their own. They are on board with the mission. Because the need for interpreting is so great now, and the languages so varied, by and large, we use a phone service to meet this need. It's wonderful to have the immediacy this affords, but my bias would be for a live, warm, body right there in the room with the mom and I.

Djibril is an African who speaks four languages: English, French, Falani, and Bambara. The latter two are dialects of many of the 18 West African nations. He told me that in Mali, his country, it's customary to be given several first names. One can alternate them at any time. When we first met, he used the name Mamadu.

I speak some French, but when a mother is having trouble, or when she is pumping for a baby in the NICU, I call him. On one particular night, I stayed late to help a mother latch her baby for the first time in the NICU. The baby, born seven weeks early, is only 1-day-old, and this will be his first feeding by mouth, as he is being fed intravenously. When possible, the first feeding is meant to be at the breast, not the bottle. This is a policy we do our best to adhere to, so a mother knows we are committed to her success. For a baby, it begins to imprint to this way of feeding, known deep in his premature yet mammalian brain. The volumes of milk and tongue movement are different when a baby is bottle-fed. The policy to breastfeed first gives the couplet the best shot at breastfeeding success, which is not easily achieved with separation and prematurity. Still, 80 percent of our moms who intended to breastfeed are discharged with their babies nursing.

This mom's baby is in Pod A, closest to the NICU entrance. Being in the front of the pod, he is more visible to any passerby. I gather the wooden screens that are five and a half feet high, while the mother and Mamadu linger and chat about who knows what. As the screens envelope her, she looks above them quizzically and speaks to our six-foot-five interpreter with the voice inflection of a question. I surmise she is asking what is going on with the screens. Of course, I am not privy to understanding the conversation, but when she begins to laugh uncontrollably, I question him. This gets him laughing as well.

His explanation to her was that in America, many mothers are shy about breastfeeding in front of others. This is so foreign to their ways, and she tells him she "could nurse anywhere in all of Africa and no one would care. It's natural." He knows this, of course, and so do I.

**

Ana is from Spain and she's a feisty, outgoing woman who dresses to the nines. I invite her one day to join a group of NICU pumping moms for a Lunch and Learn, as there was a Latina mom in the group. We offer these gatherings once a month, and moms report that they get a lot of support from both our staff and from each other as they cope with separation from their premature, and often, critical babies. As we open the meeting, one by one, each woman says her name and tells her story. I begin. When we get to the Latina mom, Ana interprets. The other mothers are patient and kind, nodding to the mother, in acknowledgement of her situation. When she's finished, I ask Ana if she'd like to say something about herself.

Wow! We learn a lot from that one lead question. Her mother breastfed all seven children, and everyone she knew in Spain breastfed. Being so much a part of her culture, she never doubted that's what she'd do. Ana arrived in the U.S. with her husband in 1998. She was 18 and pregnant with her only child. She'd read enough to convince her that breastfeeding was healthier for her baby and would promote better bonding. Ana assumed she'd breastfeed for one year, but instead breastfed for five. Today, she proudly reports now that her daughter has a 4.6 grade point average. She tells the NICU moms that human milk played a big role in her brain development. "I truly believe this is from breastfeeding. All I read was true."

Chapter Four

THE LACTATION DEPARTMENT

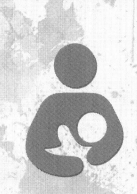

The Pilot Project: 1992

If you can dream it, you can do it.

WALT DISNEY

Hospital administrators warmed slowly to the notion of a new role and department within the maternity arena. Even in the 1990s, everyone was mindful of The Budget. Thus, the position of lactation consultant that I was offered was solely for a 6-month pilot project to test the waters. They allotted 24 hours per week. There was a caveat. The position would be PRN, *pro re nati*, Latin, meaning as the occasion arises, though we all know babies need to eat around the clock.

My first office was adjacent to the Mother-Baby unit which allowed staff to routinely stop by as I was settling in, letting me know who they thought should be seen first. Even Renee, the housekeeper, made a point to tell me she was worried about some mom in room such-and-such who was ready to give up nursing. I finally awarded her a lapel button that said, *Ask Me About Breastfeeding*, because she found herself in so many breastfeeding conversations with the mothers. "Those talks just embarrass the heck out of me, Chris," she'd tell me repeatedly. Yet, she availed herself to them nonetheless.

This accessibility to the maternity staff made it easy to gather together a dozen staff members to round out the department's first breastfeeding support team. They were eager to provide help to mothers, and learn more about breastfeeding themselves. On a practical level, there was much to do to: educate all staff, including the docs, develop forms, and explore what it would take to receive the coveted designation given by UNICEF that affirmed a hospital met a set of gold-standard criteria for breastfeeding support. In fact, in those 6 months, we did get as far as a letter of intent to receive the designation. It would be another 22 years before we reinvested in that goal and achieved it.

Three months into the pilot project, there was a glitch. I broke my ankle roller skating with my sons on the uneven blacktop of our neighborhood schoolyard.

Two days later, I had a call from Joan, a nurse and member of the breastfeeding support team. She'd been asked by the manager to assist the wife of the medical director of obstetrics. Like her husband, this new mother was also an obstetrician. While my colleague tried unsuccessfully to help the baby latch, the mother quipped, "Is breastfeeding just another one of those lies we tell our patients?" That, my friends, is exasperation talking.

We're mammals, yes; sucking is instinctual. But for many couplets, there is a learning curve for the process. Breastfeeding doesn't always come "naturally," and by this, I mean easily.

I didn't want to squander the designated time for the pilot project and returned to work using a walker. In the end, I submitted a report of statistics I'd collected for the hospital administrators. They unanimously approved establishing a lactation department, with an overwhelming "yes" coming from the OB medical director, whose wife we were unable to help.

Chapter Five

MORE MOTHER–BABY UNIT ENCOUNTERS

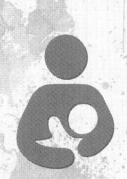

Lifesavers
Engaging the Postpartum Staff

Tell me and I forget. Teach me and I may remember. Involve me and I learn.

BENJAMIN FRANKLIN

Researchers have analyzed both the cost-saving and life-saving value of human milk. Many were astounded to learn that if the guidelines for breastfeeding set out by the American Academy of Pediatrics were practiced in the U. S., it's estimated over 900 *lives* would be saved *each* year. We're not talking the developing world here.

Over the years the maternity nursing staff has been quick to cut out articles from newspapers and magazines to share with me if they were in any way relevant to breastfeeding. It may be about a mother sharing her milk via the Internet, or a new health benefit identified for the baby. It often sparks an animated conversation, and I've appreciated these discussions and the transparency of the staff. We are all learning to be better caregivers.

In the summer of 2006, I received copies of the story from several nurses about 16 people who ventured a 100-mile journey from the Dominican Republic to Puerto Rico in a homemade boat in search of a better life. On the first day, they were already adrift, discovering their compass didn't work. They'd gone through all the food and water within the first three days. Distant cruise ships didn't see their frantic waves for help. Among the group of eight women and eight men, was a lactating mother who'd left her 1-year-old behind in the Dominican Republic. On the fifth day, mouths parched, she thought to offer her sister a few moments of suckling from her breast. In turn, the sister took milk in for her and deposited it in her sister's mouth. They both reported that they began to feel better immediately. For the following 9 days, she offered her breast milk to all passengers for brief moments. Her fellow refugees dubbed her the "Little Angel of the Sea." Her sister concluded they survived on "prayer and her sister's breasts."

More recently, in 2015 another story came out of New Zealand. A woman, with an 8-month-old at home, set out to run a 20K race in a forested area of her country. The woman, admittedly not familiar with the forest, was lost for 24 hours. A helicopter spotted her and rescued her. While she had an energy bar and a small amount of water, she attributes her well-being to drinking the milk she hand-expressed from her breasts.

What touches me are the conversations these stories elicit among the nurses. (They veer off the education I'm usually trying to convey about breastfeeding assistance and documentation on the Mother-Baby unit.) There's the sheer improbability of survival, and then the gross-out factor for some, many comments about these. But also questions about why a mother would ever have left her 1-year-old in the first place, or how so little milk would keep them hydrated. Sometimes the articles came from nurses who have shared with me privately that they struggle to support breastfeeding on the unit. It's foreign to some of those who opted to formula-feed their infants many years prior. But these stories provide segue to explore their thoughts and feelings, and I see in most of them the will to do what is right according to the research. And that is a good thing. In fact, it's all I can ask. I am never more pleased as when I see the staff in action, giving the moms the time and the support they need to be able to breastfeed. I still believe, as has been said, that people don't care how much you know until they know how much you care (T. Roosevelt). The time spent with staff has been time well-spent.

Dadancy

When life descends into the pit,
I must become my own candle,
Willingly burning myself
To light up the darkness around me.

ALICE WALKER

I met Dadancy while I was a nurse on the Mother-Baby unit in the early 90s. She is a bright young woman and very receptive to learning about how to support the breastfeeding mothers, though she herself is single. She is a good nurse, skilled and compassionate. It has to be both. Dadancy's accent has a hint of an English dialect, which makes sense because England colonized her homeland of Sierra Leone many years prior. The country has been self-governed since 1961.

Trouble was stirring in Sierra Leone as early as 1991, when the government's corruption led to economic collapse. Most of the country's professional class began emigrating, thus Dadancy's arrival in Cincinnati, where she had relatives with whom she could resettle. During the years leading up to the civil war, the government was colluding with a diamond company, and revenues from this natural resource went into the hands of the mining company, members of the government, and the business elite. It was reported that 94% of the citizen were victims of the violence.

Dadancy and I spoke of the war, though these were hard conversations for her because she knew some of the victims firsthand. By the late 90s, she decided to return to her country to aid as a nurse. I feared for her life, but she was resolute. "It's what I need to do, Chris," she said matter-of-factly. How could you not admire that courage and determination? In the U.S., nursing is always ranked in the top five most respected professions. She has earned this respect.

While events in her country dominated some of our conversations, she also taught me about birth practices in Sierra Leone. Most women return to the home of their parents in the latter stages of pregnancy and give birth there. If a mother births at home, traditionally, the attendant makes sure the baby touches the ground as he or she births. Dadancy says this is how the earth herself greets the little one. Additionally, it roots the baby to their birth home and makes it less likely that they might leave the family later. (I return to thoughts about that conversation when I reflected on why three of my own four children live hundreds of miles away. Perhaps I should have had a homebirth, on a dirt floor!) Breastfeeding, of course, is the norm. Yet, it's not uncommon for others to share in nursing the baby, generally other family members. In part, Dadancy says this frees the mom to rest because it's expected that in the early weeks, the baby be held constantly. It's an oddity for her to see our babies whisked off to the nursery (before we closed the newborn nursery) laying in the pram for hours unattended aside from feeding and diapering.

I do not know what happened to Dadancy once she left for Sierra Leone. She left us before the influx of so many West African immigrant patients. But I think of her fondly when I care for someone from Sierra Leone.

Erica

She is So much More than
a Sickle Cell Diagnosis

Sickle cell anemia is a hereditary disease affecting about 100,000 Americans. The odds of acquiring it are 1:500 for African Americans. With sickle cell, the red blood cells clump in the veins and cause severe pain and permanent damage to the bones and every major organ. When the pain is severe, they are said to be in crisis. When my friend Erica was born, the life expectancy of someone with the disease was 14. Now a person can live into their 40s or 50s, but she tells me that someone in her support group is over 80.

We hadn't talked in four years. She must have changed her cell phone number. I was taking a trip down memory lane, looking at old photo albums, and came across her picture. She's looking directly into the camera–dimpled, serene smile. Something stirs.

I'd picked her up that day in late afternoon. Quinn, her long-time beau, dad to Ennaja and Eenaya, helped her down the steps. She was a little unsteady, but managed. Erica always manages. The sun was warm and bathed us on this particular June day. She was dressed in her best skirt and multi-color print blouse with her straight brown hair pulled back in a ponytail. The clip belonged to one of the girls. She was 34 then; the girls, 9 and 6. I had asked her to say a few words at the retirement reception for Dr. Jeanne Ballard, a neonatologist and primary physician covering our normal newborn nursery. She cared for both of Erica's newborns.

In 1993, when I was first board-certified as a lactation consultant, Dr. Ballard approached me saying she was interested in the field of lactation. Our collaboration lasted until 2007.

And then there was Erica, at times debilitated with a sickle cell crisis, age 25, yet breastfeeding her firstborn through it all. I don't recall the exact number of times she was in crisis during the pregnancy, nine admissions come to mind. She was so happy to be pregnant, and now, so happy to be a mom; happier still that Eenaja carried only the trait, not the disease.

As we drove to the retirement party, she gave me an update on the girls. She was worried about her youngest. With Erica's increasingly frequent hospitalizations, and time at home spent sprawled on the couch, Eenaya, her youngest, was showing signs of anxiety: trouble sleeping, bad dreams, and reluctance to leave her mom to go to school. She was in a good school environment, with supportive teachers and staff who know the family story. It is the same inner-city Montessori school where I'd sent all four of my kids. No matter how she was feeling, Erica was vigilant when it came to her girls. She'd just met with the school psychologist and was trying to incorporate some of her advice.

Eenaya's birth was induced 5 weeks early because Erica's pain management by then included more opiates at higher doses, and her sickle cell crises were double in frequency compared to the first pregnancy. The perinatologist managing this pregnancy was afraid to let it go to full-term, for fear the baby would be in severe opiate withdrawal within a matter of hours. Birthing prematurely, it was protocol that she be admitted and followed in the newborn ICU. But two days after the birth, Erica made her case and convinced the team to transfer her baby to be under

Dr. Ballard's watchful eye. She knew Erica. She knew her firstborn. Erica trusted her. And she knew Dr. Ballard understood her commitment to breastfeed. Amazingly, Eenaya had minimal withdrawal, only some tenseness to her body and fretfulness managed by skin-to-skin holding and nursing. She was a calm baby within 96 hours. Erica did her best to drop down to one opiate again, and manage her medicines around Eenaya's feedings to have the least amount of narcotic transferring through the milk to the baby.

Eenaja nursed for 15 months. Despite Erica's many hospitalizations in the baby's first year of life, Eenaya nursed for 9 months. This was a remarkable feat and one for which she was rightly proud. Throughout this three-year period, I saw the girls at least once a month. She was faithful to stop by the office and show them off after her doctor appointments. Erica might have had a medicine tweak, a blood draw, a blood transfusion, or all three. As a result of these frequent visits, these were the only babies I got to see grow up, at least to school-age. The clatter of the double stroller making its way through the outer reception area and back to my small office was a familiar sound. Sometimes we visited there. Sometimes we'd go down to the deli for lunch. Sometimes I'd pick her up at her mom's apartment, and we'd go out to eat while her mom watched the girls.

I'd say, "You are a fantastic mother. I'm so proud of you and so grateful to know you, Erica." She'd smile and say nothing. What indomitable determination she has.

The day of the retirement party, I parked as close as I could to the hospital door, and we walked arm in arm down the corridors trying to find the reception. When Dr. Ballard saw her, she was visibly moved, and reached out for an embrace. I gathered drink and appetizers for Erica as she sat talking to other lactation consultants in my department who also knew her.

When it was time for her to speak, she stood next to Dr. Ballard. Looking out on the sea of doctors and well-wishers, she retold her story. She always speaks so softly, I extemporaneously summarized with each of her pauses, to make sure everyone heard and understood the significance of Dr. Ballard's support to normalize this one very important part of Erica's life. She ended, "You're a fantastic doctor and I'm glad you were ours." I smile at the familiarity of the phrase. God bless Erica. She was gone from my life a few years, but one day called and whispered that she's been readmitted.

"I'll be up as soon as I can."

Stopping at the gift shop, I picked up some candy for the girls and flowers for her. Quinn was on the fold-out couch, sleeping. He comes up each day, once he gets the kids off to school. While he never said much to me (I don't really know him at all), I see he is gentle, faithful, strong, and kind. He took my arrival as a chance to get back to the kids. Later, he'll ride the bus back with them in tow. She was too weak to talk. I held her hand, tickled her arm, and talked about my day with babies. These are the stories she loves. She is brave beyond belief and 38. I pray for small achievements—seeing both girls graduate from high school, and marrying Quinn. I don't have the courage or wisdom to know how to pray beyond that.

With no way to contact her by phone (though I've kept her name in my cell phone's contact list for 18 years), every now and then, I stop by the hospital's Information desk and ask if she's admitted, and I'm glad for her when they say she's not a patient.

Recently, I chanced to meet a third-year fellow who has

shared in her care. She has lived to see both girls graduate from grade school and middle school. She is 42. He talks cryptically, sounds grim, speaking in hushed tones. But when I tell him of our history, his face relaxes and he's smiling, as if with me, he sees her anew, and can picture her younger self.

A year later, I stopped by the Information desk again. She's hospitalized again. As I entered the room, she lights up, despite looking quite weak. We hug and kiss, and she retrieves her phone to pull out pictures of the girls. They're homeschooled now. Eenaja will complete her GED in June. She and Quinn hope to marry in the Fall. She showed me the ring he gave her just two months prior. He'd told the family, and they were gathered at the church where he planned to formally propose, but she had another crisis and was admitted instead. Their celebration was private, here at the hospital where they've spent so much time. She updates me on her worsening condition, but says with confidence that the good Lord knows she's not ready to go; her kids aren't grown yet.

Now, 2017, I am off work, but in the vicinity of the hospital. I call in. She's a patient. I surprise her with the book, *Crowns: Portraits of Black Women in Church Hats*. She's thrilled. She's in a book club and says she may suggest it for their next book. She's excitedly looking forward to a trip to Florida in August with her mom, sister, and aunts. She's going to bring the book along since all of them are religious. I voice a concern about the heat in August, but she's dismissive. This is the second vacation she's ever had. I'm sure she doesn't want me thwarting it. Still, I worry.

I hear about Quinn's musical abilities, and she tells me she urges him not to keep his life on hold because of her. *Pursue your dreams*. She updates me on the girls, shows off prom pictures of Eenaja, and texts Eenaya and asks her to send a picture of herself so I can see her. Eenaya's silly and sends a picture of her and Erica; she's inserted a queen's crown on Erica's head. I think it's serendipitous since I'd just given her that book, but she waves it off as Eenaya playing a stunt. There is so much normal about the time we spend together, and she seems stronger than our last visit, despite her doctor saying otherwise. I help her throw her own top over her hospital gown and briefly remove her oxygen before the nurse snaps a picture of us.

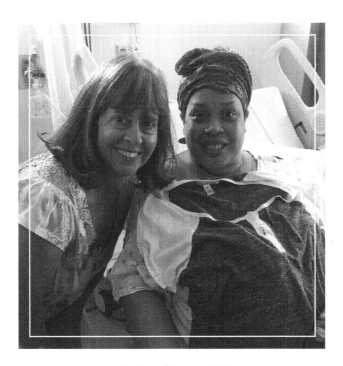

✳ *Chris and Erica, 2017* ✳

The Sweet Mom and her Humble Triple-Crown-Winning Husband

*If the only prayer you ever said in your life
was thank you, that would be enough.*

MEISTER ECKHART

Early in my career, I assisted many women who received their care from a certified nurse-midwife. We had a great team of midwives and they were instrumental advocates for establishing the hospital's lactation department. Over one particular two-day period, I met with one of their patients, a couple in room 3364. Why do I remember the room? I can only explain it because the couple was memorable. Not because of fame, as I had no idea who they were, but because of a sweetness between them that I found charming. You'd think every couple giving birth to their first would exude this. Not so. I am an observer by nature, a people watcher, and what I notice is that with some couples, it's all about focus on the baby, with only pragmatic interactions between the parents. *Warm my coffee. Ask the nurse for more diapers when you see her.* Things like these. For others, it's all focus on the visitors (or the TV). And still with other couples, I see dads sleeping a lot—more than you'd expect. Occasionally, I've joked with moms about how tiring labor must have been for Dad. And then there are dads like this man who seem enchanted with both his wife and baby, fielding phone calls to protect her rest time, and pointing out the baby's little expressions that he finds delightful. There are two other things I recall. I remember her breasts, and I remember that she was taller than he.

It was only routine care I provided. She was a little tender, needing basic assistance to create a good latch. Other than that, the visit was not that remarkable. As was typical, we talked about what to expect in the coming week at home. I did ask if she had a breast pump. She replied that she didn't. I must have anticipated a need and asked them about their insurance. It was rare in the early 90s for companies to cover the cost of a pump, but some high-end plans did include a pump in the benefit's package. Dad spoke up, saying he wasn't employed at the time and they didn't carry any insurance at all. Caring for many unemployed families, I'm sensitive to added expenses health care professionals unwittingly recommend. I had access to a free hand pump which, while not the best, would at least do in a pinch to help her through the engorgement phase in case she became uncomfortably full. (I'd recently had a NICU mom using this type of pump and expressing five ounces each session for her twins—even though I had arranged an electric pump for her to pick up!). When I gave it to them, they seemed genuinely touched and thanked me profusely. She called once the following week, then I never spoke to her again.

Only after their discharge was I told that the dad was a jockey. While we are 10 minutes from the Kentucky border, even that left me nonplussed. Then I learned more. At a young age, he became extremely successful and wealthy. Until 2015, he was the last jockey who'd won the coveted Triple Crown, that is, he'd won the Kentucky Derby, Preakness, and the Belmont races. I had to laugh. I'm so naïve. I assumed only the horse's owner won money. He could have bought her the most expensive, efficient pump on the market. I wondered if it was just too embarrassing for them to tell me I need not have given them the simple hand pump. Still, I smile as I think back to their gratitude.

Postscript

Over 20 years later, I'm at the Kentucky Horse Park with the grandkids. Ava and I saddle up in the corral on Hildalgo and Burrito. A rider is explaining that Saddlebred horses nurse the foal of thoroughbreds once they've had the colostrum because the milk supply of a thoroughbred is notoriously low. Good grief, I have to tell her my occupation. An older gentleman hears my partial retelling of the story above. He tells me he's known that man since he was knee-high to a duck, when his Daddy rigged a barrel attached to ropes and the boy, age 8, practiced racing.

The Cardiologist Who Underestimates the Organ Above the Heart

*A pair of substantial mammary glands has
the advantage over the two hemispheres of the
most learned professor's brain in the art of
compounding a nutritive fluid for infants.*

OLIVER WENDELL HOLMES

I am taken aback by the cocky intern, only months out of medical school. By and large, interns are eager and receptive learners. But he blows off breastfeeding, and intends to be a cardiologist, seemingly unable to grasp that breastfeeding lowers the risk of cardiovascular disease. The interns only rotate through the Newborn Service for one month. I'm not going to change him, and indeed, for one month, I can put up with his attitude. He's been gone for several years, but I flashback to him after the consult in room 3367.

It's their first baby. She's a nurse here; he's a cardiologist. She's in her mid-to-late 30s. It's a delight working with her and her baby. Small tweaks in the latch and she's pain-free, which is always rewarding for an LC and certainly for the mom. She attaches the baby herself on the left side and does fine. I find that most women have an easier time latching on their non-dominant side. This is what she is working to accommodate as she rotates the position of her baby. She mentions that she's so grateful to have the option of being a stay-at-home mom. Before leaving, I tell her I'll return in the afternoon.

Reentering room 3367 later, Daddy is present. Wait, no, his cardiologist persona seems to be all that has shown up. He's the antithesis of excited and quick to tell me that he's completed a thorough literature search on human milk.

"She's only going to breastfeed 3 months," he says tersely. He seems to have laid down a gauntlet before me, defying me to challenge him. I don't take the bait. I am 21 years into employment here. I've had contact with this type before. But he continues, despite my attempt to ignore his comments.

"There's simply no evidence that breast milk is beneficial after 3 months."

Mom seems to be ignoring him as well, as she notes how long her baby's fingernails are right from birth. Then, sliding the side of the diaper away from his body, she tells me he's pooped.

"Would you like to change the diaper?" I ask him, anticipating the answer that I indeed get. As I wipe his baby's bottom, I mention that she might want to discuss breastfeeding duration with her pediatrician.

"I already did," her husband pipes in. I'm struck by how much one can know about the heart with all its complexity, and so little about the organ above it that, in fact, expends more energy when lactating than the heart or even the brain, as it preforms something so vital for the survival of the species over the millennia.

We move on and discuss what she might experience over the next three days as her milk comes in full force. She lives in Hyde Park, a neighborhood with a strong La Leche League presence. I give her this support group's number, 513-357-MILK, suggesting that she may want to reach out to them.

I hope she finds her footing and her voice, does her own lit search, and does as she pleases in three months.

The Farmer's Great-Granddaughter

She tells me—I'm 71 old
grown wheat, helped raise cattle all my life
seen livestock birth, and death up close.
Waited out rain, waited for rain

can't tell ya how many
farm animals I've seen born,
then nuzzle up to a teat
to drink right after

by God,
never would have guessed
no baby'd do the same –
never occurred to me

cried like a baby myself –
first at the birth, next at the nursin',
most beautiful thing
I'd ever seen.

Postscript

Family and visitors tend to engage in conversation with ease
while I'm in the patients' room, affording an opportunity to
encourage their support, learn their story, dispel myths, make
connections, and occasionally win them over to be more
supportive of breastfeeding. It's touching to hear the stories
that tell me someone's been amazed. This particular great-
grandma was intimately familiar with birth and breastfeeding
as a farmer, but was flabbergasted and in awe when she saw
her great-granddaughter nursing.

When Weaknesses Collide

Lessens in Humility

---

*Life is a tapestry we weave day by day with
threads of different colors, some heavy and
dark, others thin and bright, all threads
having their uses. The stupid things I did are
already in the tapestry, indelible, but I'm not
going to be weighed down by them 'til I die.
What's done is done; I have to look ahead.*

ISABEL ALLENDE

MAYA'S NOTEBOOK

I may have been more laid back,
had I not begun the day
with an innocent new mother—
discovering her low birthweight baby
had never fed in the 17 hours since birth.

I may have been more generous in attitude
had it not been for the color tattoos
glaring across her chest and arms,
which I normally ignore,
but today, found annoying.

I watch her feed her 3-day-old,
a nibble, a pause, a short burst of sucks,

now long pause–mostly comfort nursing,
not eating, yet she proudly tells me
it's her best feeding since birth.

The room has a chilly edge,
enough to make babies feed poorly
since they spend energy keeping warm,
shutting down for other activities–
like eating.

I suggest she raise the thermostat
but she complains she's already hot.
I may have been more patient
had she been willing to defer her needs
to his needs.

Returning later that afternoon,
I may have looked less alarmed
had she not been so blasé
when she said she *skipped*
his last feeding due to visitors in the room.

Poor feeding, no stool in 24 hours,
significant weight loss –
with all the tact I can muster,
I suggest after the breast she offer an ounce with a cup,
not just the one-fifth ounce pumped.

I purposely avoid the word formula,
which doesn't flow easily from my lips in general,
but I already know she considers it taboo.
In retrospect, I should have asked
for a blood sugar instead.

My intent to page the resident,
as I was leaving, was to give him an update
and ask that he check in on them in a couple hours,
but that wasn't needed –
she'd called him to the room herself.

He didn't want to walk in the room blind.
He knew she was upset.
"No one else had said her baby wasn't feeding well
and what does the room temperature have to
do with eating anyway?"

I may have been less inclined
to roll my eyes at the doc,
who was patting my back for catching
the poor-feeding infant just that morning,
while the following morning I am reading his order:

"Please do not have Chris Auer see this patient.
They have a personality conflict."
Oh, brother, and I thought
I was just providing gold-standard care –
trying to prevent another dehydrated newborn.

I could have been more considerate and
anticipated her reaction.
Ya, I blew it.
But did he have to immortalize it on the first day
of converting to electronic medical records?

Salt and Pepper Shakers

A Grateful Teen

---

*A poor widow came and put in two small
copper coins, which amount to a cent. Truly I
say to you, this poor widow put in more than
all of the contributors to the treasury; for they
all put in from their surplus, but she, out of
her poverty, put in all she owned, all she had
to live on.*

JESUS

BIBLICAL PARABLE

In the spring of 1999, the maternity units converted to an electronic medical record. No more paper charts. But the day prior to this transition, I walk onto the Mother-Baby unit and am pulled aside by a nurse. She tells me that she has tried to get a new little 2300-gram (5# 1oz) baby to the breast at 9 o'clock without success. She asks if I will I see that patient early, but adds, almost as an afterthought, that the baby had *fed all night*. With this added detail, I feel it buys me some time to first see at least one mother-baby couplet being discharged by late morning. Forty-five minutes later I enter room 3366 and greet a weary, but smiling 18-year-old. The baby is not in the room.

"Congratulations on your little one," I say, "I hear he kept you up last night eating. You've gotta be tired."

"Yes," she acknowledges, and then offers this telling piece of information, "he sucked once at two and twice at five in the morning." There is pride in her voice at this sense of accomplishment.

Oh, my God, someone has documented how long she tried to feed ("all night"), not how long the baby actually fed, which I surmise was not at all.

"And where is he now?" I ask in the most casual manner I can muster, while sirens are ringing in my head. He is slightly preterm and 17-hours-old.

"He's getting his circumcision," she responds.

"Would you excuse me?" I ask calmly, stepping out of the room. Upon shutting the door, I am literally running down the hall to the treatment nursery, which is the furthest locale from room 3366.

As I'm opening the door, I see the obstetric resident holding the limp baby up in mid-air, saying, "I don't know you guys. I don't feel good about circ'n this kid." The pediatric interns look up at her from the computer around which they are huddled. They seem unfazed.

"No, you shouldn't," I interrupt. "He's 17-hours-old and has had nothing to eat." And it was settled without argument, as I grabbed a bottle of formula, a dropper, and a bottle nipple. As I streak back down to the mother's room with the baby in pram, I see the nurse and ask her to get a stat blood sugar. I make a token attempt to help her latch the baby who showed zero hunger cues, before moving on to supplementation. We normally would not let a baby born early and this small go this long without an effective feeding. Formula offered by the dropper just dribbles out the side of his mouth. Over the next five minutes, with all the years of feeding experience behind me, I can only get him to take seven milliliters, a teaspoon and a half, now by bottle.

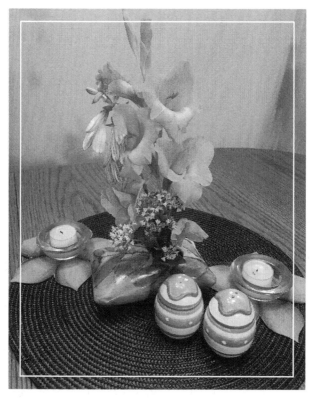

* A teen's gift *

The nurse returns with the glucometer and asks me to get his blood sugar because the pediatrician is in a delivery and he hasn't answered his pager. She says she doesn't want to get in trouble obtaining this blood work without an order. A normal reading on the first day of life would be at least 40 mg/deciliter. His sugar level isn't even high enough to register on the glucometer, which will read as low as 20 mg/d. He is whisked off to the NICU, while I assist the mom with using an electric pump.

It took a few days before he is diagnosed with an unusual endocrine disorder, pan-pituitary, that would be treated with daily injections for the rest of his life. Symptoms include a persistent low blood sugar and a micro-penis. Had I not walked into the nursery at that very minute, and the resident proceeded to place him supine on the board where circs are performed, she would have stopped the moment she opened the diaper. This baby's circumcision would have been delayed anyway.

The baby spent some time in the NICU, and over the first week, Mom worked hard to establish a good supply. She is brave and keeps her hopes positive as she absorbs the news of her child's condition. He eventually begins to learn to bottle-feed while only having minimal success with breastfeeding, despite her diligent attempts that began well before the bottles.

On the day of his discharge, she brings me a gift. It's near Easter now, and I open a cute set of pastel salt and pepper shakers in the shape of eggs. Aside from thank-you notes, over my 25 years of working with breastfeeding families, I've only received three gifts. One was from a doctor, another from a doctor's daughter. These little eggs mean so much coming from this teen mom. For 18 years, they have graced my kitchen table in the Lenten/Easter season.

St. Vincent DePaul

I am done with great things and big things
with great institutions and big success.
And I am for those tiny, invisible, molecular
moral forces that work from individual to individual
through the crannies of the world.

WILLIAM JAMES

There was a study published several years back, exploring why women didn't follow the advice of their WIC nutritionist. Bottom line: the suggestions weren't realistic for their personal circumstances. I thought about that study when local physicians were discussing what they could do to decrease infant mortality in our region, where the rate is twice that of the national average. During Grand Rounds, a neonatology fellow presented an update and reviewed the recommendations, including placing babies to sleep on their backs and in a separate bed.

I'd spent five years in a volunteer capacity for Saint Vincent DePaul, a charitable non-profit that makes home visits, helping people meet very basic needs, such as rent, clothing, food, furniture, fans, medicine, and electric bills. My assigned area is the most densely populated poor area of Cincinnati. The average age in Winton Terrace is 17. An earlier study found the area to have the most incarcerated males. There are children everywhere. So in the aftermath of the lecture, I raised my hand and shared my experience of this work.

In those 5 years, I'd only seen one bassinet in an apartment, and only one crib, which incidentally wasn't used because there was no mattress. I concluded that it was so much more important to address what is safe sleep from the perspective of what is achievable for the parent. No sleeping in a chair. No sleeping with a sibling, placed on the back to sleep, and no exposure to cigarette smoke. (Yes, this means smoking mothers may have to change shirts in the course of a day.) And finally, can we do anything to help them initiate and continue to breastfeed, especially in those critical early months when babies are most prone to SIDS?

Discharge education cannot be about spewing a checklist of do's and don'ts to parents. It seems critical that it begin with what's in the home, what's achievable, what the family resources are, and who the mom's support system will be, especially at night. I am convinced that we are missing the mark when this conversation isn't taking place while she is pregnant.

On Saturday, I go in to see a mama before she's discharged. From the chart, it seems as though breastfeeding is going pretty well. I note that there has been no supplemental formula given. Generally, I sit to talk, but as I did, she makes a funny face. "Is there something the matter?" I ask.

"Well, I'm kinda in a hurry because I have an appointment at my apartment at one o'clock with someone from St. Vincent de Paul. I'm getting baby supplies." It's already 12:45 pm. There is no way she will make that appointment. I know the volunteers who are making visits that day, and am able to call them and ask them to delay their visit. The mom becomes a sea of calm once the time pressure is off.

More recently, I am volunteering again in that neighborhood, but in a different capacity. I'm at the grade school helping kindergarteners learn to read. On the following day at work, I meet with two different mothers who happened to live in the neighborhood. "I was just there at the school yesterday. Do you have any school-age kids?"

One has a third grader, the other a preschooler. One mom's baby is in the NICU, the other has never breastfed before. This acknowledgment of working in their neighborhood school seems to help us connect. The one mom who was vacillating about continuing to attempt breastfeeding became more animated and said she did, in fact, *really* want it to work, and asks for more help. Meeting mothers where they are matters.

The Father who said NO

---

*My husband is a pivotal anchor in
my life. His influence encourages me to be
independent and take risks.*

PADMASREE WARRIOR

The nurse is asking me to see a mother who has not had *breastfeeding* designated as her feeding mode for the last two days. I proceed to her room. The mother tells me that the daddy doesn't want her to breastfeed. It's their third child, and she'd wanted to breastfeed the first two, but abided by his wishes. This time, she says she *really* wants to breastfeed this baby, but she has not begun. He enters the room as we are talking. It's an awkward middle to be in, and I think quickly about how to address his concerns.

"Mom tells me that you'd rather she not breastfeed the baby," I begin. The pause I allow is only met with silence. "If it's because of breastfeeding in public, I've had other people tell me they're uncomfortable with this. She could offer a bottle when you're out, no problem." He shakes his head to say this wasn't the issue. I pause, waiting for him to fill in more detail, but he remains silent, stoic even. I wait a bit longer before beginning again.

"Some dads feel left out when they aren't able to help with feedings. I just want you to know that you can start offering a bottle in a few weeks. Again, he shakes his head as if to say, *that's not it.* I ask him if he can articulate his concern. "I just don't want her to do it," he replies. This stops me now. If a person is unable to mine his own thinking process or the gut reaction to breastfeeding that brings him to the conclusion of "No, you can't really get very far in a conversation."

"Hmm, I wonder how you two will figure this one out?" The question hovers, perhaps too close, much like his presence in her life. "Sometimes when two people disagree on something, they let a third somebody decide." (I'm sure he's thinking I want to make their decision, but that's not where I'm headed.)

"I wonder if you should let the baby decide. If she's not interested, then there you have it. It's not going to work anyway."

He neither protests nor agrees. I take that as a passive yes (knowing it may have been the opposite) and continue. "Listen, she's already 2-days-old and just had a bottle 30 minutes ago; she's not going to nurse while I'm here because I leave in 40 minutes. So, when your daughter is hungry, Mom's going to have to either try to latch on her own, or ask the nurse for help. Would you mind if I just showed her how to position the baby before I go?"

"Whatever," he responds. Mom has not said a word during this mostly one-way conversation. My back is to him as I slide the baby in a football hold, taking care to keep her weight off Mom's incision. He walks out in less than a minute, as Mom calls out repeatedly, "Where you goin'? Where you goin'?"

She is sobbing now, shaking her head, saying she just doesn't understand. Nor do I. I get her tissues and acknowledge that she's in a tough situation, and that I don't feel qualified, nor is it appropriate for me to advise her. She nods her head in understanding. Hating to leave her in this predicament, I give her our department number and a few basic instructions. As I head toward the door, I pause, turn to her, and say, "It would be a shame, but you could consider offering your breast once or twice a day, when he's not around."

Frankly, when I leave, I'm angry at him. I doubt she'll go against his wishes, and wonder what else she's stuck with doing or not doing simply because of his opinion. Maybe they have an otherwise good relationship. Who knows? Breastfeeding could be a singular blip on the radar of how they process decisions, or maybe not.

The Californian
Birth Plan

Serenity Now!

GEORGE COSTANZA
SEINFELD

In the past 10 years, I've noticed that written birth plans are less in vogue here in our hospital. In part, this may be due to midwives, sadly, no longer delivering babies at our institution. In this region, there is an extremely low rate of natural childbirth. Attendance at natural birthing classes is down, while use of the epidural for anesthesia is at an all-time high. But in the distant past, birth plans were common. Nurses warmed to them slowly, not having previous experience with shared decision-making. But staff did adapt. They found it helpful to know a family's expectations, and would do everything within their power for them to have a wonderful experience. Still, staff came to view lengthy birth plans with skepticism. The longer the plan, the more likely some felt Murphy's Law kicked in, with hopes seeming to veer off course. This was not data, mind you; just gut feelings informed by some staff experiences.

In 2011, a patient and her husband, newly relocated from California to Ohio, ask for a Silent Birth, in a dimly lit environment in their labor room. This is a method of birthing advocated by L. Ron Hubbard, founder of Scientology. While there is no scientific data to support it, he claimed that any spoken words are recorded by the baby and mother's reactive minds and can have negative effects on them both. The family's written plan is not elaborate, but the team gathers for a simulation so that they can prepare for the expected and emergent scenarios that might occur for mother or baby in which good team communication and rapid response would be essential. They have done their homework. All staff are prepared to participate should they be on-call or assigned when the mother goes into labor. This includes: neonatologists, neonatal fellows, neonatal residents, charge nurses in the NICU, staff nurses in Labor and Delivery, obstetricians, obstetric fellows, and residents. This is no small matter.

Our lactation team is also informed that she wants to exclusively breastfeed her firstborn. I'm not surprised. Anything else would be counter-intuitive. The big day is here, and she is admitted in early labor in the middle of the night. By noon, she is fully dilated and ready to push. The room has remained very dimly lit, per their request, and ever so silent–initially. At this stage, the soon-to-be mother projects the only sound emanating from the room, slinging expletive after expletive, before, during and even after the birth, as her baby is being laid against her chest, skin-to-skin. These are the first sounds he hears, while (perhaps) not understanding.

Her active labor is less than 8 hours, short for a first-time mom. I am told by the Mother-Baby nurse to wait until the end of the day to see her because, like all mothers, she is exhausted. Only, most mothers with birth plans are asking for the lactation consultant as they are being wheeled into their room. I wait three hours, and go in to introduce myself. For all I know, she may have breastfed by now, but this is not the case. The baby is making familiar mouth movements, searching for food. The dad says he's been rooting for the past 30 minutes, and had done so off and on since the birth.

"I am way too tired to breastfeed. Just give him a bottle."

How quickly the best-laid birth plan is tossed out the window. There is no convincing her that we can hold off longer to give her more rest, deferring his needs to hers, or that she could nurse lying on her side. Dad can rock him; hold him skin-to-skin as well.

"Just feed him, just go on and feed him." Still, we had attended to her every wish with precision.

God grant me serenity.

The Giggling Dermatologists

Being at ease with not knowing is
crucial for answers to come to you.

ECKHART TOLLE

It's Saturday and I swing into room 3363 to check on the mom and baby; the nurse has told me they've been asking for me. I announce myself, and wait to be invited into the room. Dad hops up from reclining on the couch as I enter. They are all smiles. I know ahead that they are dermatologists, though I don't know how far along they are in their training. I acknowledge a friend they may know who works in the department, and they beam, saying they love Pam, my oldest friend's partner. They just seem to love life and exude enthusiasm. They share their birth story, and are pleased with how breastfeeding has ensued over these first 12 hours of their full-term baby's brief life.

I provide the teaching as they listen attentively and give them my pager number to call when the baby is showing signs of hunger. The page comes a short hour later. I return, and we prepare to feed. Examining her breasts, I note the small red area on the tip of each nipple. She says she thought a little pain was to be expected. It's only a "3" on a scale of zero to 10, she tells me dismissively. The baby's mouth is not the root of the problem, a normal palate, a tongue that extends like a serpent. I ask if she'd mind if I attached the baby on my own for the first side, then she can do the second side. She is more than accommodating.

Her baby is actively rooting and on she goes. "Oh, my goodness," she exclaims as the baby sucks away.

"Are you in pain?"

"None, but her suck... now it makes sense."

The dad is hovering in delight. "You know how we told you the baby had already breastfed three times?"

"Yes," I say, and I can tell, there's a pregnant pause in the air, and wonder what's coming next.

"Well, I think she'd never really fed at all." They chuckle at this admission and the innocence of their mistake, and all is well.

I meet them in the very same room three years later. It's their second birth. I, who had a central role after their first birth, have been set aside. She has experience under her belt now. She breastfed her daughter for a year and doesn't ask for help with her son. They don't need me. This is good. The grandparents arrive with the big sister, and they are delightfully distracted, giggling away with their toddler, as together, they count the toes and fingers of her new baby brother.

Chapter Six

THE TRUTH ABOUT NEONATOLOGISTS

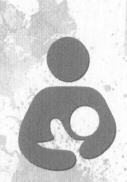

Jeanne
First Physician-Colleague

---

*A hero is simply someone who rises above his
or her own human weaknesses, for an hour, a
day, a year, to do something stirring.*

BETTY DERAMUS

I met and collaborated with a neonatologist, Dr. Jeanne Ballard, from 1992 until her retirement in 2007. Her reputation as a breastfeeding advocate was solidified when she established what is now called the Center for Breastfeeding Medicine. This outpatient breastfeeding center was initially held at The University of Cincinnati Medical Center (UCMC), and was established through a grant from the March of Dimes. In addition to my work as a lactation consultant for in-patients, I worked with Jeanne in the first three years of the center's opening. Some would say we flew by the seat of our pants. And if one is referring to our records, they were primitive compared to the electronic records and templates of today's standard. But, we knew our patients. We both cared deeply about them, their babies, and their breastfeeding outcomes. It was a gift to have someone of Dr. Ballard's reputation who shared my passion. I will always owe her a debt of gratitude for that, and for her friendship.

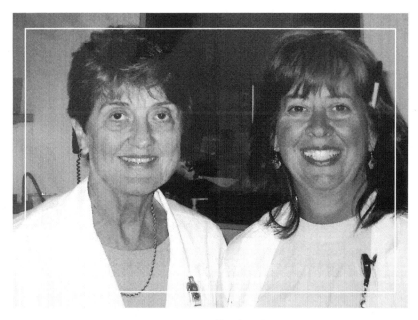

∗ *Dr. Jeanne Ballard and I.* ∗

Jeanne is likely best known in international circles for developing the Ballard Gestational Assessment, a tool that identifies key physical markers of an infant's anatomy to determine his gestational age, that is, how many weeks along the mother was at the time of delivery. This was taught to and performed by residents around the world who were assessing babies without the use of ultrasound to estimate age and due date.

We learned a lot from each other. I learned a lot of science from her, as well as how to think outside the box to solve complex breastfeeding problems. Jeanne, 11 years my senior, has said that I provided her with her initial lactation education, even after breastfeeding four children. When she was a resident and having her first baby, it was her obstetrician who told her how to breastfeed. *Begin with nursing 1 minute on each side. At the next feeding, 2 minutes per side, increasing in 1-minute increments until the baby is nursing 10 minutes per side.* We both laughed and sighed when she first told this story. Of course, it was the obstetrician, not the pediatrician, who would get the calls about sore nipples. Back in the 60s, their inaccurate understanding was that the nipples had to "toughen up," and nursing in gradually longer time increments (but not too long) would prevent soreness. We now know that short feedings with a poor attachment to the breast is the usual culprit, not long feedings with a great latch.

In 2002, Dr. Ballard and I published a paper together about the incidence and assessment of tongue-tie, and the impact for the mother and baby when the skin tag is clipped. It remains the largest study to date on this still somewhat controversial subject. Our work at the outpatient center included improving many poor latches, but it also included tongue-tie cases. I've included two cases later in this book.

Mike
The Irish Neonatologist

Mike, in his mid-30s, was the youngest neonatologist in the group of six who oversaw the care of babies in the NICU in the mid-90s. He was a cheerful Irishman, married, and had one child. Mothers appreciated that he was often mindful of the work of pumping, and generous in expressions of encouragement, especially to those moms with very tiny babies, who had a Herculean task to maintain a supply for 6-to-8 weeks before there was even a possibility they could attempt direct breastfeeding. Mike was spontaneous in compassion, unafraid to embrace a weeping father or mother.

When his wife's name appeared on the maternity unit's census one morning, I went to their baby's chart to review how feedings had gone since the birth. She was 15 hours old and full-term, and it was documented that she'd fed once at 9-hours of life. Looking further back in the record, I saw she'd had a brief 8-minute pushing phase prior to the birth, likely the cause of her disinterest in feeding. I was not worried. Babies that birth this quickly tend to still have some of the amniotic fluid in their system, and are often spitty and initially disinclined to eat.

Entering the room, Mike greets me warmly and introduces me to his wife. After the congratulatory fanfare, I comment that it looked like their daughter had figured out the job of eating at 3 in the morning. They stare at me, mystified. I bring the chart over to their eye-level so they can read her record. Mike lets out a sigh of understanding.

"Fifty minutes?" he questions. "That was how long we tried, but she didn't eat at all."

For me, however, this was the precipitating event that allowed me to convince the manager to introduce a breastfeeding assessment and documentation tool into infant charts so nurses could describe the effectiveness of a feeding more comprehensively than charting minutes alone allows.

Henry

The Neonatologist Who Needed to Help His Wife Pump

He describes using a hand pump, swinging his arms in a heave-ho motion, recalling the ache of his upper body from 30 minutes of pumping his wife every three hours over the course of two days, until the milk flowed like the Nile River. "It was torture," he sighs and chuckles.

Dr. Akinbi's wife is also Nigerian-born. They met in their native land. Meeting was a miracle alone, in a population of over 174 million residents speaking 512 indigenous languages. The country houses one-fourth of the entire population of Africa. Speaking the same language was the other miracle.

The couple arrived in Chapel Hill, North Carolina, where Henry completed his fellowship in neonatology. When he accepted a position in Philadelphia, his pregnant wife was well into a master's program in pharmacy, thus the decision was made to live in separate cities until her education was complete. He traveled back for the birth of their daughter.

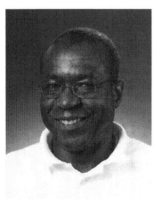

* Dr. Akinbi *

Initially laboring at home, she arrived at the hospital too close to delivery to receive anesthesia. Henry describes the 2-day postpartum stay as uneventful. Their daughter breastfed fairly well, he recalls. Once home, a full milk supply did not arrive as expected on day of life 3. Their daughter wailed, the cry of the forlorn, not understanding why her hunger wasn't abated. About 108 hours after the birth, her milk finally came and so did extreme engorgement, clogging the milk flow like a backed-up drain. Henry spoke by phone to the breastfeeding consultant who was nearly an hour away. "Buy cabbage and wrap the breasts..." he trails off.

"This was her advice, Chris. I didn't believe it—but I was willing to do anything. I did exactly as she instructed."

When milk rained down, the ritual of trying to extract milk with a manual pump began because she was returning to her academic program within a week of the birth. Even after breastfeeding this now-happy newborn, there was plenty of milk available to quickly fill their freezer. Though it was a shaky start, they made it through this event exclusively breastfeeding. Their daughter continued to nurse for 16 months. I am not surprised that this physician-dad remembers the details of those early days after birth as though it were yesterday. He rubs his arms after demonstrating how he used the hand pump. Muscle memory still recalls the ache.

By the second baby, they were in Cincinnati. I was with them after this birth. I'd never have known by the calm demeanor of Mom and Dad that there was any residual worry about milk supply or flow. He tells me that this has influenced his approach when seeing breastfeeding mothers on the maternity ward. He has more empathy, knowing that it's not always easy. While his wife was able to get through this early crisis without supplementation, he listens thoughtfully as moms express their various concerns. If they are discussing quitting from exasperation, he gives them leeway to supplement briefly rather than stop nursing altogether.

Sometimes this permission lessens some internal pressures, and the next morning, he finds at least some of them still nursing.

Understanding his pumping crisis helped me understand why he left me a two-page hand-written letter after he readmitted a 4-day-old baby, born to African parents, who had not been feeding for a day due to his mother's extreme engorgement. She had breastfed her first over 2 years with no problems in Africa.

Despite knowing a hand pump's limited efficacy, he closed his letter with the following query; "Couldn't they have at least been given a manual pump?" I suppose he thought if he could go through the labor of manually expressing milk for his wife, any man could.

Laura

A Neonatologist Who Became a Champion

I am careful as I write my story of this neonatologist; she is someone I admire. I want to do her story justice because it is a stellar example of how personal experience impacts the trajectory of one's career pursuits. It was not an easy journey, but as Laura says, "We all have our crosses, don't we?"

I met Laura shortly after she was a newly hired neonatologist, moonlighting part-time in our NICU in 2002. Her story began earlier though when she was in Kentucky, her husband assigned to Fort Knox, paying back his dues to the Army for subsidizing his education to become a surgeon. Their son, Jackson, was born there in November 2001, 4 weeks early. Four weeks doesn't seem like much when she'd helped babies survive who were born 16 weeks early. But Jackson was exceptionally sick, not having well-developed lungs. Additionally, he struggled with pulmonary hypertension, a condition resulting from the failure of normal transition in blood circulation after birth, causing the blood to shunt from right to left. We are talking life and death, and as she well knew, Caucasian males fare worse than females or non-Caucasian males. In NICU lingo, they were referred

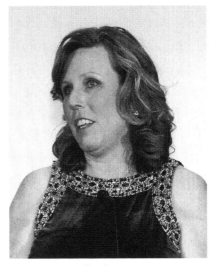

✳ *Dr. Laura* ✳

to as WWM's: wimpy white males. This did not help boost her confidence in a happy outcome.

It's hard enough to pump when you are separated from your newborn, worse yet when you are trying to push the image of a burial out of your mind. Laura pumped with a vengeance, this being one of the few things she could do as hints of ECMO intervention floated around her. The ECMO machine takes the blood from the baby, oxygenates it, and then returns it to the body using an artificial heart. While this intervention was averted, Jackson was on the ventilator for a full week, and remained an NICU patient for two weeks.

Her supply kept up with his needs, but barely. Once Jackson was home, she began in earnest to exclusively breastfeed him; after all, by this point he was considered a full-term baby. At the first follow-up appointment, he hadn't gained. We look at these babies born at 36 weeks with much more caution now, knowing that even when above seven pounds at birth, as he was, they can take longer to feed effectively. The pediatrician recommended she pump after each nursing and feed the milk back to him. We call this triple duty. It is exhausting: breastfeed, pump, bottle-feed, and repeat. Anxious to grow him, by 3 months, she introduced cereal. It wasn't the solution, but mothers, even neonatologists, get creative when they're trying to solve a problem their child is having, even when everything in their training says it's not a good idea.

After her maternity leave, she was commuting two hours to Cincinnati, to moonlight in our NICU, staying with her Cincinnati aunt who was watching Jackson while she worked. By this time, she was consulting with Dr. Ballard, known for her work in the field of lactation. There was no miracle cure to boost her supply, but amazingly, she breastfed for 6 months. Even 14 years later, she recalls seeking my advice, particularly sad when she compared her supply to some of the high-supply NICU moms. I've found all comparison to be diabolical. You only have your life story; it seems best to embrace it. She remembers that at one point I said that the grass isn't always greener; these moms, too, have their struggles with oversupply. Still, when she meets with NICU moms with ample supply, something tugs inside.

When her son was 15-months-old, her surgeon-husband was deployed four months to Iraq with the first wave of soldiers. Back for a mere three months, he was deployed again for another seven months. Nine months after his return, they welcomed their second son. Malcolm was full-term and breastfed well from the beginning. The fear of eking out an adequate supply prompted her to begin pumping daily right after she was discharged from the hospital. One ounce, one ounce, one ounce. She persevered. With the return to work, her boys remained at Fort Knox, while FedEx shipped her milk on dry ice in the *Graeter's* ice cream coolers she went through like water. Her feat? He had only her milk in the first year of his life.

Laura continued to pump for 15 months, as Malcolm's first exposure to cow's milk was disastrous. Her husband called up to Cincinnati one day to tell her he was in the middle of a chemistry experiment; he was busy mixing small aliquots of cow's milk to her milk, titrating up as their son tolerated it, and eventually, he did.

In the midst of this experiment, our hospital entered into a national Human Milk Project, largely focused on how to get more human milk, and specifically more of mother's milk, to very premature babies. Laura was naturally drawn to, and has participated in the project for over 12 years. In addition, she has been an integral stake-holder as the neonatologist-team member for our Baby-Friendly certification.

Laura traveled the necessary distance to work for 3-and-a-half years, with two children and a husband awaiting her just south of Louisville. Sometimes the journey you commute from where you are to where you want to be begins with surrendering to what is. Laura has lived that with grace and style. I hope she is proud of her accomplishments.

Jean

The European Neonatologist Who Pressed for Donor Milk

Jean, a neonatologist from Luxemburg, speaks with a deep, baritone voice and heavy accent. It was not uncommon for him to stop in the middle of rounds, wash his hands, and pick up a crying baby. He would bring their ear near his lips and begin talking softly to them.

"There, there, there. What's the matter? You're okay. Come on, come on. Calm down."

With his voice so deep and soothing, these efforts were remarkably successful in calming most babies within a few moments. I've never seen another physician offer this comforting gesture.

In 2004 and 2005, he was a strong advocate of introducing pasteurized donor milk into the NICU for the smallest babies when their mothers were not yet producing substantial amounts of their own milk. But, as I learned after numerous meetings with the group of neonatologists, they agree on very little. In early 2006, as medical director of the nursery, he suggested I survey the mothers themselves to gauge how they would feel about its use, and whether it would affect their commitment to pump. The results were overwhelmingly positive, at which point he recommended I apply for a grant to pay for the initial 125 ounces. It took until November to secure a grant from Ohio La Leche League. As the supply ran low, he simply said, "Place the next order."

And just that quickly, we were able to eliminate the risk of exposing the gut of very low birthweight infants to the foreign protein of another mammal. We are indebted to him for this.

For years, he was the primary physician at a high-risk infant clinic, and as such he continued to follow these NICU graduates. Parents bonded to Jean. They had no doubt this was a man who cared deeply and was committed to their child. For that alone, he was the recipient of their affection and admiration.

Steve

The NASA Consultant Who Believed in the Power of Skin Contact

*

Steve, the attending physician, begins bedside rounds with lighthearted air, asking if anyone has a joke or story to tell or something interesting from the news. He begins. He's been trolling around the Internet and found Wikipedia. In his sage-like manner, he explains that it's a new resource of information, a little like an online encyclopedia, with the caveat that anyone can edit or add to the body of knowledge. This could create some question of veracity, but it is so novel that Steve is clearly enamored despite the fact that it doesn't jive with his scientifically rigorous upbringing in academia. Next, a riddle shared by the pharmacist, and then we are on to the serious matter of keeping babies alive.

We move from crib to crib, the 15 of us inching along like hungry beggars in a bread line, waiting for scraps of information and crumbs of insights and logic to explain away why one baby or another is or isn't getting better.

Arriving at the incubator of the latest admission, I see she's under 2 pounds, thus considered very low birthweight, which is a flag that her mother will be asked to pump milk whether she intended to or not. The resident spews detailed numbers of blood counts and resuscitation measures. The respiratory therapist chimes in with stats of oxygen saturation and tube placement. The pharmacist delivers her assessment of whether she should be on a long or short-term course of antibiotics. The social worker provides a family history: mother with osteopenia imperfecta (OI), wheel-chair bound, an independent spirit, husband inappropriately affable with a history of traumatic brain injury, and a supportive grandma.

Nutrition will be discussed next. There is pressure to start feedings, since, as Steve reminds us, this 26-weeker has been drinking amniotic fluid for months. He's resistant to my bias to wait for mother's milk. Everyone knows mother's milk is safest, but it's 2004, and they haven't quite grasped that formula in this fragile gut can pose its own counter risk. He reluctantly defers to keep her NPO, nothing by mouth, for another 24 hours.

Now the pressure transfers to me to get milk. I withdraw from rounds to visit her room—only no one has explained OI to me. It's not that I'm alarmed to find her naked; it's a maternity ward, after all. But her mother and husband are chatting away with her as though it was a pajama party and they'd been gabbing all night. But someone has forgotten to wear pajamas and it seems it's gone unnoticed. Besides this, and more alarming, she is laying horizontal in bed, with room to spare. This is the plight of those with OI, short stature, and fragile bones. It would have been nice to be prepared for what I encounter but I have more pressing concerns right now.

She has indeed started pumping, and points to her three tablespoons of milk sitting on the bedside stand, an enormous amount for this tiny, but well-endowed woman. Wide-eyed, she's grinning over her accomplishment. I proceed with 20 minutes worth of education, still her nude, Grandma and new Father taking it all in; he with his off-handed comments, she with her well-thought questions, confidence, and optimism. In my mind's eye, I step back to people-watch, as I often do in airports and playgrounds. She lets her daughter take full charge, never interrupting. It's no stretch to conclude she grew up being well-loved. Briefly, even I have forgotten I am in this conversation with three people, all of whom are oblivious that someone is lying crossways naked in the bed.

It's on to paperwork now: insurance forms to authorize a breast pump for home. I notice it's asking for her height. In all my years in lactation, this is a first. Good grief, what do they need that for? It's a breast pump. I am too embarrassed to ask her height. I look at the bed, figuring its width to be the size of a yardstick and jot down 28 inches.

In rounds the next morning, I mention my encounter and the dilemma of asking or guessing her height and Steve cannot contain his laughter. She's got to be close to 32 inches, he's remarking, and I wonder why that is the only oddity he found in the whole story. You're going to quibble over four inches? I doubt that the insurance review board would believe either number.

**

We learn after X-rays that the baby had multiple fractures while in the womb. She, too, has OI. Everyone is so careful when handling her. The parents visit daily despite living an hour south. Dad continues to say wildly inappropriate things, which staff overlooks because of his injury. She is making tons of milk. She has an amazing body and we are all happy for her. It's one of the few bright spots in their story. The weeks pass and the baby has outgrown her incubator, and is now in an open crib. Mom sees that other mothers are behind screens, holding their babies skin to skin.

She wants this too. She's yearning for it, sitting in her wheelchair, milk dripping from her breasts like the tears she doesn't cry.

***

On morning rounds, the nurses are in a tizzy. The night-shift nurse allowed Daddy to place Mommy in the baby's crib to cuddle. They thought it looked ridiculous to others, and who knows if the crib could actually handle that added weight? Who cares? She's over-the-moon happy with this new connecting, as any first-time mother of a preemie would be. Discussion ensues, but there is no conclusion on rounds. There is no policy prohibiting a parent to be in the crib with her baby. It had never come up before. However, Steve's specialty is skin, the body's largest organ. He believes in the power of touch. He does contract work for NASA, and knows and understands fetal development on earth, as well as in zero-gravity outer space. He does not see what the problem is, but he's worked with our 87 nurses long enough to know not to ignore their concerns. And so, it continues for three days before he comes up with a creative alternative. Leave it to Steve. He calls in Infection Control, gets their approval, and devises a mat for the floor where the baby is carefully transferred by the nurse and respiratory therapist to her eagerly awaiting bare-chested mother, screens surrounding them. The baby is stable there, and Mommy is in bliss.

****

Over time, the baby needs more support than we can provide, and she is transferred to Children's Hospital in the early morning hours, and with her go the family's social problems. We process, in silence, past the empty crib on rounds.

*****

We meet again two years later. She is thrilled to have carried this second baby to 32 of a normal 40-week pregnancy. Steve is aware of the birth. Though not on service this particular month, he bids them congratulations. The baby will be normal stature, no osteopenia imperfecta. Daddy is slapstick happy. The stay is relatively brief, but in its course, I see that she is adept at handling her baby, agile and skilled in infant care, even from her chair.

******

Returning from a weekend outing at a Kentucky lodge, my husband and I make a bathroom stop at McDonalds. And there they are, happy family of four, plus a friend. It's Sunday, and they're having a bite to eat after church. He is grinning ear-to-ear, and she appears her joyful self, eating and tending the babies in a modified stroller and car seat.

Vivek

Yoga, The Indian Neonatologist, and His Obstetrician Mother

Dr. Narendran was a new neonatologist when I first met him. Since 2007, he has been the medical director of our NICU, and an early supporter of breastfeeding. He is from Bangalore, not far from the southern tip of India. His mother, who resides in India, is an obstetrician. They are Hindu, and as such, are steeped in the tradition of yoga and meditation. In 2005, just prior to accepting the position of director, he published a fascinating paper with his mother and several of her colleagues. It was the study of the effects of yoga, stretches, and meditation during pregnancy on outcomes of birthweight and gestational age at birth. In other words, how close to full-term were these deliveries? The mothers were taught the postures (asanas) and breathing techniques (pranayama) to accompany their meditation. They began a regimen of one hour per day from the time of enrollment in the study until the birth. The outcomes for these babies were compared to a similar set of pregnant women who acted as the control group and were advised to walk 30 minutes twice per day.

The results indicated that the mothers practicing yoga carried their babies longer and had higher birthweight babies than the control group women. Additionally, the yoga practicing mothers were less likely to have pregnancy-induced hypertension (high blood pressure), a fairly common complication of pregnancy. It makes sense. Transcendental meditation is known to reduce resting heart rate and oxygen consumption.

Why does this fascinate me, over 10 years after its publication? The reasons are three-fold. First, we strongly advocate for mothers to hold their babies skin to skin for at least an hour while they visit their babies in the NICU. It has been shown to stabilize heart rate, respiratory rate, and temperature in babies, as well as reduce length of stay, help establish later breastfeeding, and improve bonding. The mothers often report a sense of relaxation while they hold their babies in this manner. While this isn't yoga or transcendental meditation, it seems to act as a stress reducer for both mothers and babies. So often these women are under stress when their babies are born premature, and cortisol, a stress hormone, would likely be high if we measured it in moms.

Additionally, another set of mothers with high stress levels are those in drug treatment programs trying to maintain abstinence. Studies have looked at ways to decrease stress in pregnancy by offering regular phone calls, counselling, and home visits by health care workers. These were not found to be effective in reducing psychosocial stresses in pregnancy. In Dr. Narendran's study with his mother, they speculated that the interventions in these studies were too focused and not holistic enough. Yoga, with a combination of mind, body, spirit, may just prove to be an intervention to reduce stress and anxiety in this subset of needy mothers. I wonder how it would affect relapse rates. I think it's worth finding out.

Lastly, we know that sharp rises in stress hormones can lower, and at times, completely eliminate a previously good milk supply. Conversely, would relaxation promote a better supply? I don't think I would have connected the dots in these ways had I not read this article by a mother-son team. I believe in the power of focused deep breaths and reciting a word during meditation. My word for these mothers and babies is *Hope*.

Noah

The Neonatologist Who Worked in His Boxers

One month after finishing his neonatology fellowship at UCMC, Noah's wife gave birth to their own preemie at another facility. He had just been hired by our hospital to be an attending physician in our NICU. Noah is easy-going and has a good sense of humor. No doubt he found irony in his circumstances as the father of a preemie.

This delivering hospital had a policy that allowed parents to board until the discharge of their baby, a wonderful option I wish all hospitals offered. Within days of his child's birth, one of our NICU nurses was sent to the same hospital for observation because her water broke. Felicia was barely 32 weeks along the 40-week journey to deliver a full-term infant. This is a particularly critical window for fetal lung maturation. About 30 percent of these babies will have severe respiratory distress. Felicia debated during her two-day stay about whether to transfer to our hospital where the Level III nursery is better equipped to handle complications.

In recounting the story once back to work, she said she was quite surprised when Noah came to her room on the second evening to listen to her concerns as she tried to process staying or transferring to our Level III NICU. He reassured her that her baby would be in good hands if she stayed. Noah told her he was pleased with the care team's management of his own first-born who was slightly more preterm than Felicia's baby at that point. She'd had no idea of his baby's birth, but after an hour of discussion, felt peaceful about staying put. With that, Felicia went to sleep.

She was awakened around 11 that evening with the first contraction. She put on her call light, and as Felicia told me the story (mere days after returning from her maternity leave), she voiced regret that she hadn't said to the clerk answering the call light that she was in labor. It was the changing of shift and she'd only asked to *see* the nurse. This discounted the urgency of her situation. Her night shift nurse didn't arrive for two hours. By this time, she was five centimeters dilated—half way to show-time. She was immediately rushed to Labor and Delivery while staff paged the on-call obstetrician and pediatrician. At 10 centimeters and ready to push, the obstetric resident asked her to pant instead, in an effort to ward off the delivery until the more experienced physicians arrived. Wits about her, instead, she begged them to get Noah. Unassuming as he is, the staff was unaware that he was a neonatologist. Knocking on the door of the darkened room, the nurse entered and began by asking, "Are you a neonatologist? We need you in Labor and Delivery."

Arriving in his boxers and socks, Noah donned a scrub gown and quickly prepped for the birth. It was 3 in the morning. Her son was delivered by the resident with Noah, who attended to the respiratory needs of the baby, with serendipitous timing. The on-call attending physicians arrived 20 minutes later.

Nine years later, she once again recounts every detail of the story as though it had happened the week prior.

"Thank God he was there."

Over time, her son improved his breastfeeding skill and she nursed him for 8 months, the same length of time she breastfed her second child, born full-term.

Noah and his family have since relocated to another state. He is remembered with special gratitude by Felicia, but also fondly remembered by more than this one nurse.

Chapter Seven

STREET DRUGS

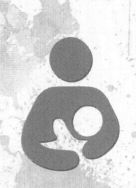

An obstetrician and I were astonished when we attend an open house sponsored by a drug treatment center. We had made the 40 minute drive in hopes of providing our patients better care. Among the myriad bits of information, we learned that previously, their earliest support group session was at seven in the morning, until they offered one at 5:30 a.m. The caseworker assigned assumed he'd have one or two early-risers attend. He was shocked when the room was overcrowded with more than 50 recovering addicts. After the session, these clients were off to their jobs as businesswomen, airline pilots, and physicians, to name a few. I wished he hadn't mentioned any occupations.

A Mother and Her Newborn's Drug Withdrawal

No one is immune from addiction:
it afflicts people of all ages, races, classes,
and professions.

PATRICK J. KENNEDY

The baby is in the midst of an all too familiar feeding frenzy. This is not to be confused with cluster feedings, when a baby feeds at frequent intervals. As she switches from left to right breast, I see her baby's ruddy cheeks and jittery body. Without bothering to read the chart, I recognize what I am seeing, having witnessed it hundreds of times. I plunge into a conversation the mother would likely rather avoid. She's been on a fairly high daily dose of methadone, 120 milligrams, since she was 4 months pregnant; prior to that, heroin. She denies relapses since starting a treatment program early in her pregnancy. I'll wait to confirm this until I read the social work consult. I've learned it's best to verify what these mothers report. I've been burnt more than a few times by believing mothers too readily. Still, my bent is to give them the benefit of the doubt.

On her weather-beaten face, I see panic rising. She's clutching her baby tightly to soothe him, but it's to no avail. "He's just hungry," she declares.

I counter haltingly, "This behavior isn't really typical. He's been nursing for two hours." I'm persuading her to see her baby through the lens the pediatricians will use. I place him on the bed in front of her and we watch him "shiver," or so she thinks. His movements are more than the sporadic startle reflex observed in all newborns. He is jittery, even when slightly swaddled.

"Maybe he's just cold."

She's desperate to interpret his behavior as normal. It *is* perfectly normal, for a baby in withdrawal.

As time goes on, the baby sleeps fitfully, never longer than in hour increments. When awake, his cry is nearly incessant and high-pitched. I open his chart and see that it's time for his every 4-hour withdrawal symptoms assessment. If the score is above an eight for three consecutive times, he will not be going home when she does. She mentions she is craving a cigarette as we review this Finnegan withdrawal assessment tool together. His score is seventeen. There is no doubt in my mind his withdrawal is severe enough, and has gone on long enough, that he needs his own exogenous micro liquid dose of methadone. It will taper as his symptoms improve. While the average length of stay for an infant's treatment is 16 days, some babies are difficult to taper and have stayed with us for nearly two months. In 2015, every 25 minutes, a baby was born in the U.S. suffering from withdrawal.

I gently broach the topic of withdrawal, and she throws her hands over her face and begins to cry.

"What will I tell his daddy?" she asks as she throws her arms up into the air.

She tells me that she has kept her own addiction and treatment a secret from him. She gets up at 5 a.m. daily, and is one of the first in line at the Indiana Treatment Center. I have no reason to doubt this. With her treatment group this early, she can get her methadone, complete her random urine drug screen, and be back in bed by 7:15, well before her boyfriend wakes. I don't get the idea that he's a frequent bed buddy, but even if it were only once or twice a week, this scenario seems peculiar. I don't ask.

"What do I tell his daddy?" The question lingers in the air.

"How about the truth?" I offer. Her reply stops the conversation in its tracks.

"Oh, that'll never work."

The Mother Who Has
My Cell Number

Before you can break out of prison, you must
first realize you are locked up.

UNKNOWN

In April 2011, I am consulting a mother who is on 105 mg of methadone. This is twice the dose I used to see when methadone first became more frequently prescribed for pregnant mothers getting off heroin. Now I see up to 175 mg, and it's not just heroin moms are getting off of; it's opiate pain pills like Vicodin and OxyContin. At 2-days-old, Emily's baby shows no significant signs of withdrawal based on the Finnegan score we use to identify NAS. His score is less than eight, which means he won't be transferred to the NICU for treatment. Still, it's standard practice to keep these babies at least three days for observation. It's Saturday, so they can't discharge the mother because her methadone clinic isn't open on Sunday; she'd have no way to get her dose without remaining a hospital patient. To miss even one dose could easily set Emily on the streets to prowl for drugs.

It's early afternoon; the attending neonatologist is gone for the day and the intern is on-call. Emily tells me she forgot to ask him some questions when he was in her room during morning rounds. I write out her questions to help her remember when he arrives Sunday morning: "What pediatrician should I see in Indiana?" The second question is the one she is intent on.

"How can I get off methadone quickly, but safely for the baby if I'm breastfeeding?"

We discuss this latter question, but she insists she can wean herself quickly, as if she knows all about the process. She complains that the treatment center just wants her money. Emily's convinced that being for-profit, they want her on methadone indefinitely. She is sure they raised her dose during the pregnancy for the same reason. I try to explain that higher doses are commonly needed because a mother's blood volume increases during the pregnancy; so many mothers feel on edge and uncomfortable, indicating the current or pre-pregnant dose is insufficient. But no, it's because they want to make more money, she says definitively.

I have met the team at Emily's treatment center. They are proactive with pregnant women, giving them priority for program admission, even when they can't pay. They sincerely want these babies born healthy. Addicted mothers-to-be are required to be in a weekly support group. The caseworkers actively encourage breastfeeding and try to help the moms keep relapse at bay, knowing they are at higher risk of losing custody if they give birth with a current or recent positive drug screen. And, of course, there is risk of death from overdosing on street drugs. One case worker agreed to lead a 5 a.m. support group. He made the sacrifice of a very early shift for the sake of these clients. I just don't buy that they are in it for the money. I counter Emily's beliefs about the program by telling her about my experience with their staff, but she doesn't back down from her original opinion.

Trevor's Finnegan scores are low, averaging six, partly due to his high tone—his muscles are stiff, not relaxed as expected of a newborn. He occasionally has multiple sneezes, and his cry, though infrequent, is high-pitched. If this doesn't worsen, he'll be discharged with her on Sunday, after she receives her morning methadone.

Before I leave, we reviewed a pamphlet together about signs of worsening withdrawal symptoms, where to get a breast pump if needed, when to call her pediatrician, and how to reach our outpatient lactation consultant. I think she's equipped with the support and information she'll need at home.

There is something sweet and engaging about this young woman nursing her baby in room 3359. The next morning, as I leave church, I call the unit and asked to be transferred to Emily's room. I want to know how the conversation went with the doctor. She asks if she can call me back because Dr. Steve is there with the interns examining her baby. I give her my cell number. This neonatologist is on the board of an in-patient addiction recovery center in Cincinnati, the only one that allows a mother to bring her children with her if they are under age 12. He is knowledgeable and compassionate.

She calls me 30 minutes later and tells me he explained in more detail the risks of rapidly weaning off methadone. I am relieved to hear she understands. While she can't set up her follow-up pediatrician appointment on Sunday, one of the docs gave her the name and number of a practice near Emily's home where Trevor can be followed. These visits are typically within two days after discharge. She assures me breastfeeding is continuing without difficulty. Her breasts are feeling heavier and she notices that the milk is changing color: again, good signs. His Finnegan scores have remained low.

At discharge, he's only lost 5 percent of his birthweight. This is also a good sign, since babies in jittery withdrawal are burning more calories and tend to lose more weight than this. He's 61 hours old at discharge and goes home exclusively breastfeeding. Mom seems to understand that breastfeeding lowers the risk of withdrawal in babies, but does not prevent it and close follow-up is essential, both from the breastfeeding angle and the NAS potential. If symptoms worsen at home, babies are readmitted for treatment.

I work Monday through Wednesday the following week, then leave Thursday with my husband and two college-age sons, who are on spring break. Our daughter in Arizona is joining us as well, all converging on Columbia, South Carolina to attend our son-in-law's deployment ceremony, and to meet our 13-day-old grandson, Nate, baby brother to Ava, age 3. It is an emotional trip. Our son-in-law is the lead medic responsible for 496 guards headed to Iraq.

We return to their house, exhausted from the first day of activities, and my cell phone rings. It's my former patient. Trevor is now 9 days old, only 6 days younger than my new grandson asleep quietly in Aunt Jen's arms, as I walk out to the deck to speak in privacy. Emily seems wound up. Her mom's car has broken down, so she missed getting to the clinic for both her Saturday and Sunday doses. I'm not sure what she wants from me, but I listen and try to brainstorm a bit, but she doesn't seem to have options. She's screwed. Yet, sometimes these moms are quite resourceful, so who knows? I think, maybe she'll get her weekend doses after all. Her calling me after discharge on my personal phone crosses a professional boundary that I unwittingly encouraged when I'd given her my cell. But I'm on the line now, so I ask how Trevor's doing and she says he's just fine. "How was his weight at the first doctor visit?"

"I didn't make it."

"Another car issue?" I ask.

"No, that doctor wasn't on my insurance plan," she says, with an air of utter nonchalance.

"So he's been home 6 days, and no health care provider has even laid eyes on him?"

Her life, like so many addicts, is chaotic. I tell her I have to call the hospital's discharge coordinator, and will leave a message for her to call Emily first thing Monday so they can find a pediatrician on her plan. The guideline calls for a breastfed baby to be examined between day of life 3 and 5. This is even more important for a baby at risk for NAS.

By Monday, when we are on our way back to Ohio, Emily calls again. She has weaned abruptly, not just the baby off the breast, but herself off the methadone.

"Are you kidding me? Just the opposite of what the doctor recommended?" I ask, unable to contain my agitation.

"I'm doing good. I can't afford it anyway." She tells me the methadone program allowed her to receive her dose at no charge while she was pregnant, but not so now. At seven dollars per day, it adds up. (Not much more than the cigarettes she's buying daily, I think to myself.) *Gratis* doesn't jive with Emily's earlier accusation that the clinic is in it for the money, but we don't discuss that.

"You've stayed clean since Saturday?" I'm sure my doubt rings in her ears as we speak. She assures me she has, but I'm skeptical. I think it's unlikely that she could be doing this well with no opiate for 72 hours. I'm flustered enough that I don't even remember to tell her how to deal with the engorgement she must be experiencing.

"I'm just gonna go on record as saying I'm totally against this, Emily. This is a disease of relapse. You're playing with fire. And abrupt weaning can make the baby sick. How is Trevor? Did you make it to the doctor?"

"That nurse called from the hospital yesterday and I've got two possible pediatricians."

"But no appointment?" I don't know if she's hearing worry or disapproval in my voice. I have a bit of both.

"Not yet. I went to WIC yesterday though." Personally, I worry that Emily is simply avoiding the system, but I hear no crying baby in the background to confirm my suspicion that he's withdrawing.

"And you asked for formula?"

"Yes." I heave a sigh of relief that she has something to offer Trevor.

"So... the nutritionist *saw* the baby?"

"Yes. I told her I'm gonna take him to my old family doctor. I think that'll work out."

Emily goes on to say how much formula she gives, and how often, and I inquire about his wets and poops, and ask exactly where Trevor is as we speak.

"Sleeping in the kitchen," she replies.

I don't bother to ask why Trevor's in the kitchen, but do ask if Emily's on the same floor as the kitchen. She is. Still, I hear no crying. I tell her I have to get going and that I can't receive any more of her calls. She says she understands.

It's 2 o'clock in the afternoon. I remind her that she should call and make the appointment with the family doctor, pronto. I want to be forthright with Emily, so I tell her I'm going to let our hospital's social worker know what's going on. She doesn't panic as many mothers would, simply saying, "Yes, I know."

I don't know why she's called. Support? A life-line? Someone she thinks might hold her accountable? But I'm the breastfeeding consultant, not her case worker, and this is not a breastfeeding mother. I've no idea what happened to either of them. As a hospital-based lactation consultant, we have no built-in follow up with moms who decide to stop breastfeeding.

Denial

---

*I am convinced that virtually every
destructive behavior and addiction I
battled off and on for years was
rooted in my insecurity.*

BETH MOORE

---

*(Though the U.S. is only 4.6% of the world's population,
we consume 80% of the prescription pain killers. There
are more heroin deaths in our Midwestern area than
elsewhere in the U.S. Vicodin, Percocet, and methadone
are the three most commonly abused substances. Heroin
is rearing its ugly head again, only now it can be laced
with the deadly drug: fentanyl. In his book Dream Land,
Sam Quinones, tells the tale of a small Mexican town,
where heroin is "selling like pizza." North of the border,
Americans are the desperate recipients.)*

It's 5 p.m., really, time for me to leave, when I receive a page
requesting a consult in the Recovery Room. A mother sits up in
bed, IV and baby in one arm, blood pressure cuff and another baby
in the opposite arm. There is something about her appearance
that makes me swing by the nurse's desk and ask if there is anything
I should know ahead of time. "Her tox was positive for opiates",
the nurse said.

"Opiates or methadone?" I ask. (Methadone is itself an opiate,
but the toxicology drug screen is specific enough to distinguish
them.)

156

"Both," she replies.

Her two slightly preterm infants are both rooting for food as I approach.

"Your babies are darling," I begin, as I introduce myself. "What did you name them?" She tells me she is going to let her daughter do that. She's 7. Okay, whatever. I've heard stranger things. They're rooting, and since they've already been exposed to the opiates via the placenta, and since colostrum is present in small quantities, I decide to assist her in latching them on. Once they attach, I tell her I know her urine is positive for opiates on admission. She opens her mouth and pulls back her lips and cheek to show me clearly rotting teeth.

"I've got to get this tooth taken care of. I took a Vicodin for the pain," she explains. "I know I shouldn't have." She qualifies, "It was an old prescription, though." It's plausible, given the black hole that is her dental picture. I remind her that the social worker is going to have to get to the bottom of it, and she nods, nonplussed.

The next day, I'm back for additional assistance. Mom is moving well for post-op day one after the cesarean-section. I see one daughter has slightly high motor tone, more so than her sister. Her arms are flexed, which alone is not unusual, but I can't pry them to extend. This is abnormal, and this evidence of high body tone is often the first symptom we see in withdrawal. I take her to the baby bed to change her diaper, and while there, I hold her forearms to lift her to a sitting position. Normally, a baby's head would lag back as this is done. This baby is as stiff as an over-starched shirt. In fact, I likely could pick her up and she'd hang from my fingers as if swinging on a monkey bar. This early symptom doesn't bode well for her immediate future. I ask if the social worker has been in yet.

"Yes," Mom says, a bit too quietly. I open the computer to read her note. The social worker is still investigating the mother's claim of a current prescription for the opiate. While this is still up in the air, I continue to help her breastfeed.

By day 3, one baby has been transferred to the NICU for withdrawal treatment. I stop the social worker on the unit. Yes, she's gotten to the bottom of it. The babies' daddy left the mom for her brother's girlfriend, and she's finally admitted to using street drugs off and on before the birth to "cope." There are tears and remorse and a phone call to 241-KIDS, Children's Protective Services. Our department policy says I can't continue to support breastfeeding because the relapse was so recent. Most research concludes that mother's milk helps to minimize withdrawal symptoms, and even if a baby has to be placed on methadone, those who receive mother's milk tend to have a shorter hospital stay. The pharmacist says it's not because of the methadone in milk, as it's not substantial, but that there is an opiate receptor in milk that likely aids in the calming effect. Breastfeeding also helps with bonding, likely eases some guilt, and may even influence a judge's decision about custody, but our policy is unbending. She needs to focus on her own recovery. Her own mom, who already has custody of her 7-year-old, will be taking on these slightly preterm, very fussy twins.

Chapter Eight

TEENS

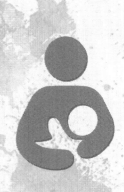

Encounters with Teens

Life is what happens when
your cell phone is charging.

UNKNOWN

---

*

I am in the pregnancy center's waiting area chatting with a mom who I'd helped with breastfeeding a few weeks ago, when a young woman interrupts us.

"I can't wait to have this baby and breastfeed again. It was the best experience of my life."

This is good PR for the mom who has delivered and is faltering in interest in continuing to nurse. I ask her how far along she is.

"Thirty-three weeks," she proudly exclaims. Seven weeks to go. I'm sure the physician's goal is to get her through these last weeks uneventfully. She tells us that she's 21 and has a daughter who's 5, who she nursed for a year. She was born 6 weeks early. She then proceeds to ask if it was okay that she added expressed milk to her child's cereal that morning because she was out of table milk. I assure her it was fine for her daughter, but ask for more details. She used both hands to squirt her milk right into the bowl, she tells us with pride in her countenance. Explaining that this kind of breast stimulation could actually trigger early labor for someone with a history of early labor, I suggest she not repeat it. She nods in agreement.

"I was already admitted a couple weeks ago with contractions, and I'm telling you it was hard to get any sleep in that hospital. The baby in the room next door cried a lot, which was making my breasts cry too."

I suppress a laugh. By this, she means her milk was leaking in response to the crying newborn.

"I finally just got out of bed and asked her if she wanted me to help her get the baby latched on, which she did, and so I got him on the breast the same way I did my daughter. That mom was so relieved, and I finally got some sleep."

✳✳

Reading the chart in the morning, I triage the patient in room 3366 to the end of the line. The baby is less than 24-hours-old and she's given seven bottles of formula with no breastfeeding documented. This makes her less of a priority than other mothers who are actually nursing. I continue reading her history. She has two other children, the first, born 12 years earlier when this mother was 14.

I make it to the room by 2 o'clock in the afternoon and after asking about her experience with breastfeeding, she tells me that she breastfed her first for 2 years.

"You were 14 and pulled that off? Wow. Nice going." She is beaming.

She proceeds to say her second, like this newborn, refused the breast. Hmm. I rarely can get to the bottom of these stories from the past: breast refusal, low supply. As best I can, I piece together bits of information and conclude it is likely that, at least for this full-term infant, she panicked and started offering formula needlessly when he didn't latch with the first few attempts. This baby is now getting acclimated to a firm, long artificial nipple, with a fast flow of milk coming in large quantities. I try to convey that healthy infants may need time to recuperate from the birth, that, a few don't even begin nursing until close to 24 hours of age, yet they go on to do fine. She seems skeptical. Now we will be pedaling backward, trying to coax the baby back to Mother Nature. In contrast, so odd that at 14, she followed an unknown stranger's advice and breastfed her first child over twice as long as the average American mother.

✳✳✳

Her baby was born at 34.6 weeks gestational age, under the weight limit for being allowed to be with her on the Mother-Baby unit. He was eating well by mouth and maintaining his temperature. It looks like it will be a brief four-day stay in the NICU. After her routine birth, we meet in the Labor and Delivery unit as she begins to express her milk. She was 12 when she got pregnant, and a few days after the birth, she'll be turning 13. She is mature for her age, which likely sounds crazy to any outsider, but I have had other

13- and 14-year-olds with which to compare her. She is quiet and always a bit disheveled looking when we are together.

Aside from her large breasts, she has the small frame of a middle-schooler. I found her to be a good listener, staying attentive to the many details of information I need to pass along prior to her discharge. Her stay after the birth is a brief 39 hours. She did not intend to nurse, only pump and offer her milk by bottle. It will be one day before an electric pump is shipped to her so we send her home with a hand pump for the interim. These are not as effective in emptying a breast, but she is returning the next day and promises to bring in the supplies we'd given her so she can pump while visiting in the NICU.

Unfortunately, she didn't come into the unit until after I left, and the evening shift nurses, only giving formula thus far, didn't know she'd been pumping, thus didn't think to ask her if she needed to pump. Mature, but not mature enough to speak up for what she needed, her breasts began to back up with milk like bottle-necked rush hour traffic.

The baby is doing so well that it was decided that if this mom and her own mama spend the night, and all went well, the baby will go home with her by early afternoon the following day. I am a fan of parents rooming-in, but I am not a fan of parents spending the night the evening immediately before discharge. They go home exhausted because they are either too afraid to fall asleep, or the baby is getting them up frequently during the night. No one sleeps, or at least no one sleeps well. When I hear of these pending plans, I advocate for the overnight to be two days prior to discharge so Mom can go home and sleep it off, especially a 13-year-old.

I meet up with the mom in the overnight room by mid-morning and find that it's been over 24 hours since she's pumped. We gather

her equipment and she turns the pump on. The bottles fill, and fill, and fill. She stops pumping once the last of the 23 ounces has been expressed. I have not seen, nor since seen, this huge volume of milk at day 4. Her mother, who has no frame of reference when it comes to human milk, is on the phone in the background, the whole time making fun of her daughter. "You should see this girl. She's a milk carton. Oh my God, this girl is crazy. What we gonna do with all that milk? I'm not keepin that in my refrigerator!"

I don't know if my "*Good job, this is spectacular,*" is enough to counter her mom's discounting comments. I have often thought of how unexplainable life can be. Adjacent to this incubator, a 36-year-old mom of a baby, conceived by fertility treatment, is desperately trying to make more than a half an ounce at a time while this 13-year-old is making six times that amount.

✶✶✶✶

She's 16-years-old. The daddy is 18 and has been given a deferment of exactly two days before he's deployed to Afghanistan. They are simple folk from a rural area. The delivery, on this Wednesday morning, was by cesarean-section. I am greeted by a room full of family well-wishers. She has requested to see me because the baby is 4-hours-old and hasn't eaten. No luck with breastfeeding in the Recovery Room. It is a difficult latch for this tired mom whose nipples don't want to cooperate with Mom's desire to breastfeed. Ultimately, she does nurse, but I can see that the piece of tissue attaching the base of the tongue to the floor of the mouth is quite short, likely impeding tongue movement and compounding the latch difficulty. It's risky to bring this up so early because, while tongue-tie is nothing to be alarmed about, it can cause a bit of a melt-down for some parents who take this as a loss of the "perfect baby." It doesn't soothe when I assure them that in an earlier era, midwives kept one fingernail long, to sever the tie if it was identified as a baby birthed.

They are young, innocent, and have so little time together with their child. When I return the next morning, a tired dad is leaving to go home and shower, and a humbly dressed maternal grandma has entered the room. We are listening as Mom says she didn't have any luck with breastfeeding after I left. "It was a struggle," she explains. She's decided to focus on pumping.

The attending pediatrician enters and discusses the tongue-tie, suggesting that clipping the skin tag, called a frenulum, may help breastfeeding. He departs with the admonition to let him know within the hour if she would like him to perform this less than 2-minute procedure.

Her mother reminds her, "I had this done for Will, remember?"

Will, I learn, is her 9-month-old brother who is still breastfeeding. Perhaps her own pumping will last as long, but for now, she will have a peaceful last 24 hours with her husband and newborn.

Chapter Nine

ON THE LIGHTER SIDE

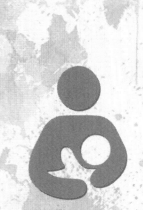

Encounters That Make Me Smile

People who never get carried away, should be.

MALCOLM FORBES

---

*

Series of titles patients have given me:

"I have to get off the phone. The lactitionist is here."

"The breast doctor's here. Gotta go."

"Get out of the bathroom, it's the boob lady."

"Are you the lactationist?"

"Uh-oh, the breast lady." (This said smiling, while giving the baby a bottle.)

"The lactating nurse is here."

"Are you the boobologist?"

"What's a lactation consultant?"

"The doctor's here. ("No, I've told you, I'm not a doctor.") It's the lady who says she's not a doctor, but she's the only one who knows what she's doing around here."

✳✳

She greets me with telling familiarity, and I know I've helped her before. She's genuinely happy to see me and proud to show off her baby. "Third girl," I muse.

"Lucky mom!" she says. She's quick to snatch her purse, rifle around, and pull out a professional packet of pictures. She's had the one and three-year-old professionally modeling for JC Penny. I learn it pays pretty darn well. She's so good-natured, so industrious. I marvel to myself, but worry: three babies in four years and she is only 21?

We catch up on trivia followed by the routine discharge education all mothers receive. Birth control is on the list because today, I'm her nurse, not the breastfeeding consultant. I broach the subject and she tells me what hasn't worked in the past.

"Have you ever considered abstinence?" I query.

"I'd be glad to try it, Ms. Chris. How does it work?"

I explain, mirroring the same nonchalance as her retort. She draws back, and says assuredly, "Ohhh, that's not gonna happen." And we both burst out laughing. Of course, it's funny and concerning. After a bit, we hug and part. I leave, thinking I may be seeing her next year, but hoping it won't be the case. Indeed, I didn't.

✳✳✳

While hearing accents from over 77 distant lands, it's the southern drawl that I find most endearing. They are as close as 10 minutes across the Ohio River. I listen and smile inside as my Kentucky neighbors speak their *y'all's and yes ma'am's.*

Spending time with one such mom, I observe: Mom nursing, 6-year-old son quietly reading on the couch, 3-year-old daughter cuddling momma in the bed. Now this 3-year-old's crystal blue eyes widen and brows furrow, as she registers the event she's witnessing a mere foot away.

"Mama! Whaaat are you doooin'?"

"I'm feeding your baby brother his milk, sugar, just like I fed Joshua and just like I fed you."

She doesn't miss a beat and shoots back in her southern twang. "That's just nuts!"

✳✳✳✳

I'm attending my first International Lactation Consultant Association conference in Atlanta in 1996. Though I came alone, I've been set up to room with two women who know each other, and were willing to bunk in the same queen size bed. During the first evening's reception, the three of us are approached by someone from the conference planning committee.

Dr. Gene Cranston-Anderson has brought her research assistant, and they are asking if we might accommodate another roommate.

The young woman with the dimpled cheeks smiles shyly as we meet outside the hotel room door. Inside, she speaks rapidly, exuberant with enthusiasm about participating in the conference. She looks to be about 21. Kylie hops in bed after her bedtime rituals. As she rolls toward me, she asks quietly if she could share something personal.

"Of course. What's on your mind?" I ask. She curls up to a sweet childhood memory as she wraps herself in the blanket.

"I haven't slept with anyone since I was a child in Japan," she confesses. "I remember the night my mother told me I was going to have a baby sister. I was 7, and it seemed like such wonderful news to fall asleep to, but then my mom and dad said I'd have to stop breastfeeding. My heart sunk. I loved that ritual of nighttime snuggles and nursing." She seems to drift off now, in a reverie of her own. This conference brings it all back. "I feel lucky to have had 7 years in their bed, and I missed it for so long."

"Where did you sleep after that?" I ask. I'm thinking she's been dispensed to the hinterland, some room far from her parents.

"On a mat of my own, at the end of their bed."

✳✳✳✳✳

At this same Atlanta conference I choose to attend a session about ankyloglossia (tongue-tie), its treatment, and its impact on breastfeeding. The speaker is Dr. Evelyn Jain. She's Canadian. It was extremely validating to know that others around the world were identifying this potential obstacle to successful breastfeeding, as Dr. Ballard noted in her practice. Within the first year of the breastfeeding center being open, we noticed the problem, yet there was a paucity of research available then on the subject. Dr. Jain began her PowerPoint lecture with an anecdotal story.

She was at a window seat when she flew across the Canadian border and landed in New York's JFK International airport. Some passengers departed and new ones boarded before the final leg of the journey to Atlanta. She was joined by two 6-foot men wearing cowboy hats. They settled in for the flight. She opened her laptop and began adding notes to her lecture. Twenty minutes into the flight, the gentleman in the middle asked if she would mind telling him what she did. She explained that she was a family physician in Calgary, Canada, adding that she runs a center for breastfeeding mothers. The two men exchanged glances and grinned.

They went on to tell her they were from Texas and sold bull sperm in Europe. It had been a grueling trip and they were looking forward to getting home, when they collapsed into their airline seats in Germany. A young mother and her infant settled into the aisle seat next them. The baby was fussing even before take-off and the two men rolled their eyes at each other, anticipating a miserable flight. As the plane ascended, the baby's cries became even louder, then, just like that, he said, snapping his fingers—silence. I looked over amazed and saw she was breastfeeding. Leaning into his buddy, he whispered, "And here all this time, I've been chewing gum."

✳ ✳ ✳ ✳ ✳ ✳

I'm covering breastfeeding rounds for 12 weeks at a satellite hospital for someone on maternity leave. Entering the hospital room, the family seems familiar. Maybe she's a doctor at my other hospital. First, we chat about the birth.

"Is this your mother" I ask the mom, "or dad's?"

"They're my parents," she tells me, smiling shyly. Grandma has been speaking a native tongue to the young child in the room, and I bow in reverence toward the grandparents. The infant son hasn't eaten in 5 hours, except a teaspoon of formula given twice by Mom. We talk about what had happened during the night, and they're worried about supply because of what happened in eastern Ohio when their first daughter was born. She mentions that she'll be returning to work in 7 weeks. I ask if she works for our hospital system, and while she says no, she mentions that she works across the street at the research lab near my home hospital. So I couldn't have seen her at work, yet, still, she is familiar. I begin to undress her newborn son and she whispers to me, "Should we have our *daughter* step out during the feeding?" I'm caught off guard by the question.

"Are you going to have your dad step out?" I ask, thinking this is really where the question is headed, but she visibly draws back, and says, "Why, no."

"Then let your daughter stay. This is something that you're going to do 8 to 12 times per day. She's going to see. Let her know it's normal." And while the baby feeds, the big sister observes for a while, then she's jumping into Grandma's arms and they are reciting the alphabet in a bit of a bouncy tone.

"She's so smart," I comment, as the baby continues to nurse.

"Yes, and she's learning Spanish, too."

"So she knows three languages? English, Spanish, and was that Hindi they were speaking earlier?" I ask, looking into momma's deep brown eyes.

"Yes," she and dad answer in unison.

"Are you teaching her Spanish?"

"No, she's learning it in school," they say with pride.

"Where does she go to school?" And now the lightbulb in my head is going off. I have seen these parents at my granddaughter's preschool in the vicinity. Suddenly dad has his phone out and is showing me class pictures and videos of the girls, and laughing at the irony of it.

I tell them my cousin became engaged at the Taj Mahal, and again they laugh and tell me that even though they're from India, they'd never been there.

****

Interpreting Baby Behaviors
a Different Way

Crying would be pointless if mothers weren't
genetically programmed to respond to it...The
mother, the father, even strangers feel moved
when a baby cries. The immediacy of crying is
"logical," adaptive behavior which natural
selection has favored for millions of years,
because it promotes the survival of the
individual.

DOCTOR CARLOS GONZALEZ
PEDIATRICIAN, AND AUTHOR, KISS ME!

"He's so lazy." Actually, he's just in his sleepy phase.

"I don't want him to be dependent on me." Hmm, it's hard to be on-call, but that's the nature of the newborn mammal. We don't hop up on all fours or trot off like horses after birth.

"My mom says not to pick her up when she cries." What's your heart say?

Chapter Ten

ENCOUNTERS AFTER DISCHARGE

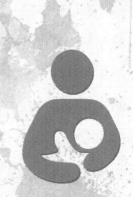

The Mother with the Dangling Nipple

By perseverance, the snail reached the ark.

CHARLES SPURGEON

The mothers coming to the outpatient lactation center are referred by their private pediatricians who know Dr. Ballard well. She had credibility before her interest in lactation, and this helps pave a trusting relationship with many pediatricians in the city. This trust is important because in 1995, when the center opens, many physicians are skeptical of this relatively new profession of lactation, in part, because they may be insecure from their own lack of training in lactation management in medical school, as well as some uncomplimentary encounters with moms who they thought too zealous. Some women seemed like extremists to the physicians. Many physicians had grown so comfortable with the use of formula that they were taken aback by mothers who insisted on avoiding it when baby was gaining fine, but mom was, for example, put on antibiotics for mastitis. Weaning was commonly recommended for inaccurate reasons. In the early 90s, only a rare physician considered unwarranted formula to have untoward consequences on the baby and on breastfeeding.

Our very first patient at the center is Amy, a beautiful, chestnut-haired, first-time mother who desperately needed help before leaving for a week-long business trip with her husband. As she comes in with her son, she comments that in the future, she would not be able to say that breastfeeding doesn't make your nipples fall off. It is said so lightheartedly, all three of us laugh—that is, until she removes her bra.

We'd never before, nor 20 years since, seen the type and amount of damage done to this highly sensitive body part. It would be nearly three weeks beore latching could even be attempted. Red and raw, but not bloody, partially dangling from the areola, these nipples are every new mother's (and lactation consultant's) worst nightmare. The human race would have never survived if this were at all *typical*. For 48 hours, Amy electrically pumped only the least affect side, while hand-expressing the most damaged side, in short intervals. You can't apply a butterfly bandage to this tissue, though the butterfly is often used in place of stitches for wounds that aren't too deep on other body parts. Dr. Ballard prescribed *Bactroban*, an antibiotic ointment, and over time, even with the use of the electric pump to protect her supply, the wound healed. Amy is such an amazing trooper.

Upon her return visit with the baby, she tells us how she pumped religiously while out of town and stored the extra milk with dry ice. She was successful with breastfeeding once her nipples were healed and the baby's tongue-tie resolved. Tongue-tie was the culprit and was easily fixed in a few seconds by a scissor snip procedure performed by Dr. Ballard.

As Amy said, "I just knew I had to persevere." With each subsequent baby, and there were seven, Amy returned for assistance and support. She was really the expert well before her last birth of twins, but it seemed the bond that was formed with Dr. Ballard over those 11 years was strong, and the visit with the twins may have been only a security blanket.

In 2007, I invited Amy to speak at Dr. Ballard's retirement party. Although she was unable to make it, she sent along a lovely tribute and a beach picture of those darling seven children.

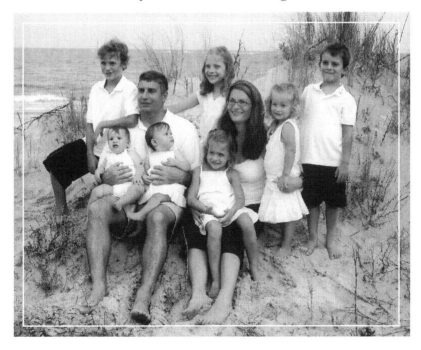

* Amy's 7 children *

On Poverty

A Tale of Two Mothers, Miles Apart

Breastfeeding is a natural "safety net" against poverty. If the child survives the first month of life (the most dangerous period of childhood), then for the next 4 months or so, exclusive breastfeeding goes a long way toward canceling out the health differences between being born into affluence... It's almost as if breastfeeding takes the infant out of poverty for those first few months in order to give the child a fairer start in life and compensate for the injustice of the world into which it was born.

JAMES GRANT

PAST PRESIDENT UNICEF

*

When seeing babies at the outpatient breastfeeding center, my first impression had never startled, but when Monica came in with her 4-month-old, my mind began to race with worry. The baby was alarmingly failing to thrive. With prominent eyes and sunken cheeks, her features were not unlike starving babies in ads for developing-world relief efforts. Monica had been to the pediatrician the day prior, and he had recommended she set an appointment at the center. Now I was glad we'd gone ahead and squeezed her into the schedule. There was nothing from the phone call that warned me it was an emergency. She simply said her pediatrician recommended that she come in because the baby wasn't gaining well. That was an understatement!

As Monica told her story in person, we knew that she, indeed, understood the gravity of the situation. The baby had gained well at every check up through the 2-month visit. At that point, the next visit was scheduled another two months out, coinciding with the baby's next immunization. Monica, a single mom, had returned to work just after this 2-month visit to the pediatrician.

She was employed driving a city bus during the night shift. The baby stayed with a woman in the same downtown apartment building. Monica would pick her baby up, nurse, fix herself a bite to eat, and then go to bed for the next 7 or 8 hours. For those 2 months, the baby slept in her bed and nursed intermittently as mother dozed. Our best deduction of what transpired was that the baby had begun to latch by just barely grasping onto the nipple, eking out only small amounts of milk. Meanwhile, Monica's body reacted by making less milk each day.

She was heartsick; feeling mortified that she'd not noticed what was now apparent. Monica was so proud of how initially successful breastfeeding had been but now tears streamed down her face as she recounted their story. We both felt for this mother, as Dr. Ballard gave her a box of tissues and embraced her while quietly reassuring her that her baby would soon be better. While Monica worked to rebuild her milk supply, she provided the baby with plenty of formula nutrition to boost her gradually back to the growth curve she'd fallen off. Rebuilding Monica's self-confidence as a mother would take longer than rebuilding her supply.

I firmly believe that breastfeeding acts as a safety net for infants born to low-income mothers. Monica's story reveals the wider implications of her poverty that include not having a breastfeeding support network among her bottle-feeding peers and not having a network of well-connected friends that could help her tap into lactation resources sooner. I saw another infant shortly after Monica's baby. It prompted me to reflect on the different lives of the mothers of these 4-month-olds, from drastically different environments.

**

Cindy was not a patient at the lactation center. She was the sister of a neighbor, and was in town with spouse and child, visiting from a suburb of Detroit. Her firstborn, Emily, was 4-months-old. Susie, her sister, called asking if I had time to come over and examine Cindy's breasts, as she was experiencing nipple pain that radiated into her chest wall. She'd had no nipple pain prior. While it's beyond my scope of practice to diagnose, I agreed to go over and provide a little guidance. I'd met Cindy before when she was in town. She was a pleasant, healthy woman in her late 20s, with a supportive husband who is a successful businessman.

Arriving at the house, I learn that Cindy is on an indefinite leave-of-absence from the firm where she practices law. She has a group of friends who are also breastfeeding moms. She'd begun having breastfeeding problems less than 24 hours earlier. The baby is still sleeping, and we chat before I take a look at her breasts. Her red nipples, shiny skin, and description of pain are symptoms strongly suggesting infection, likely requiring medicine before she starts feeling better. She agrees to call her doctor on Monday.

I am confident that Cindy will follow through, be treated, and continue breastfeeding Emily without missing a beat.

As the baby awakened, she begins to root, smacking her lips until she finds her fist to suck. Great, I'm thinking, I can watch her latch. I express my delight that I'll get to observe a feeding. But instead of Cindy picking up her baby, she picks up her Day-Timer (pre-smart phone) and begins to scan her elaborately detailed notes on dates, times, and minutes of each feeding.

"Cindy!" I address her, even as I snatch her little black book and close it without perusing. "Tell me you have not been keeping a daily record of Emily's feedings for 4 solid months? Look at your baby –what's she telling you?"

With that, Cindy ekes out a chuckle that explodes into a belly laugh. She realizes the obvious, and picks up her baby.

Chipping Away at Inequity

*Assume the best, find common ground,
and find human connection. If we can find
that grace–anything is possible.*

BARACK OBAMA

I am proud of the work our hospital has done to reduce racial disparities in breastfeeding. At the same time, I am well aware it's a drop in the bucket. While in our state, there is a 20 percent lower breastfeeding initiation rate among African American mothers compared to the general population, at UCMC, the rate is now virtually the same: about 80%. Still, we have a long way to go. There is more work to do to empower the mothers, to create support networks within their communities and churches, to improve the duration of breastfeeding, and to listen to what the mothers are saying, so we understand better what they consider to be supportive and unsupportive ideas and means of communicating that we health care workers, both African American and non-African American, offer.

I am proud to live in a city whose mayor set a radical goal to lift 10,000 children out of poverty within five years. Yet we all know that inequities and racial bias within the city, country, and health care system are longstanding. I was reminded of this during a conversation with an African American retiree near my age, as we exercise on the circuit at Curves.

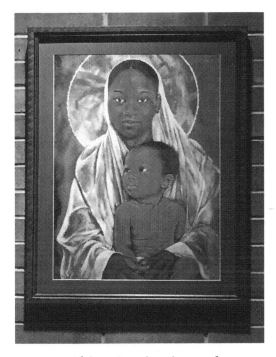

* *African American image of*
Sacred Mother and Child in our parish sister-Church *

"When we lived up north, Mya, my second, was born early and was in the Intensive Care. During my hospital stay, more than one nurse seemed to be quizzing me about what I might have done to cause her preterm birth." We look quizzically at each other as we pant away while we jog in place. At this point, I tell Caroline that I've worked at University Hospital for over 40 years, and have worked as a breastfeeding consultant in the NICU for many years.

"Over ten percent of preterm births happen for absolutely no known reasons, Caroline."

"But you know what they were getting at, don't you?" she says to me. And to be honest, I didn't, and said so.

"Well, on the last day, a pediatrician I'd never met came in. So, I finally worked up the nerve to tell him how it made me feel accused when these nurses questioned me suspiciously. He walked right out of my room, saying he'd be right back. When he came back, he said, "I'm sorry. No one will say anything like that to you again. Sometimes when a mother has used cocaine, she can have a placental abruption like you had.""

"Oh, my God. That's terrible. I'm so sorry." And I proceeded to tell her I'm a conference committee member for a Spring conference about eliminating racial disparities in breastfeeding and infant mortality. She told me that she'd read that even a college educated-black woman like herself was vulnerable to losing a child before the age of one.

"It's true," I answer, as I dry the beads of sweat gathering at the nape of my neck. Then we both pause in the middle of our routine, at a loss to explain the unfairness of it all.

She's an optimist, she says. And her 30-year-old son is too. It bothers her that he's been discouraged by the state of the country of late. She says, "I tell him, I haven't raised you to come this far, to give up now, no sir. Things will get better, things will get better."

I assure her it was good to meet her. Indeed, we met each other. It was a good encounter, and ones like this reinforce my commitment to chip away at the inequities I see and the inherent biases I must own.

The OB Chief
Who Avoids Eye Contact

Everyone has to make their own decisions.
I still believe in that.

GRACE JONES

I greet the chief resident of OB in the hallway of the high-risk inpatient unit. Her long auburn hair flows down her back like a wedding veil. Leigh's eyes, somewhat cast down, are telling me something. I'm not paranoid—or paranoid enough to think she's avoiding me. But I conclude she must be avoiding *something* with her hesitant reply and faltering steps.

I see the small bump of a belly on the young chief and tell her I hadn't heard, offering congratulations on her second child. It's May, and Leigh will complete her residency in less than two months, move south, and have this baby in the city where she plans to join a thriving OB/GYN practice. With all these wonderful new beginnings, still, she's pausing.

"Is there something the matter?" I ask.

"I can't do it again," she says with a downtrodden sigh. And I know she is referring to breastfeeding. Two years earlier as a second-year resident, I'd seen her regularly entering and leaving the Employee Lactation Room, just four doors down from my office. Leigh was busy. I was busy. We only said hello in passing.

Now she's expecting again. I wait and her story comes out, one detail at a time, like unwanted clothes still packed in a suitcase of yesteryear.

"I can't go through with breastfeeding because I can't go through another case of mastitis."

She is in the minority. Fewer than 18 percent of lactating women report breast infections. Of those who do, some have told me they felt absolutely horrible. I reply by saying, "It must have been a doozie."

"Try seven, seven in nine months."

How in the world could this happen? Women used to be given a seven-to-ten day course of antibiotics. "Was your course of antibiotics too short?" I query. But she assures me it was always a 14-day course. I jump to another idea, wrong antibiotic, perhaps the bacterium was an unusual strain. Leigh names a few antibiotics she'd taken and they are all first-line of defense meds. If fact, she tells me, with the final bout, she went to the ER pleading to be put on IV antibiotics to knock the infection out more rapidly. The ER doc must have felt bad for her, because she was allowed to go out the door the same night, IV bag in tow. This would never be allowed any layperson.

Next, I ponder the hectic pace of our Labor and Delivery unit and my mind jumps to the conclusion that she probably didn't have the time to pump regularly and thoroughly. Getting backed up with milk (usually from a skipped feeding) is a common precursor to an infection. "How often could you pump while you were on-call?"

"I pumped religiously, rarely spacing emptying longer than three hours apart."

And then I hit on the right question. "Do you remember about how much milk you typically made? It's fine to guesstimate."

Without missing a beat she says, "Seventeen ounces."

"Remind me again how long you were going between pump sessions?" I ask incredulous.

"Never more than four hours," she says matter-of-factly.

"Was that just in the final month?"

"No, I was making 17 ounces ever since I returned from my maternity leave when she was 10 weeks old."

She can see my eyebrows rising. I am known for wearing my reactions on my face, and my eyes were likely bulging in shock. Inside, I am so sad that she went through so much when there are relatively simple strategies to reduce milk supply. I am also sad that the breastfeeding training that obstetricians receive is so sparse that she couldn't self-diagnose.

"Is that a lot?" she asks.

I preface, "Did any of the other pumping employees comment on your supply?"

"All the time," she says, as the same lightbulb is going off in her brain. "Women often said that they were jealous. I just took it to mean that many people experienced low supply."

"Oh, my dear, Leigh, I wish I would have known. I could have helped."

She is not crying at my pronouncement, as I surely would have been had the tables been turned. She is stupefied that there could have been a relatively easy fix—if not before bout number two, surely for the rest.

"I assume neither your doctor, nor the ER doc, thought to ask you how much you were producing?" The question is rhetorical. To give her perspective, I tell her my own daughter pumps 5 ounces when she wants to give her 3-month-old a bottle. This is more than enough for her baby. *Five ounces.* The number seems to float like an elusive feather between us as she settles into this news.

"When did you stop pumping?"

"Right after the last bout—it broke me, Chris."

"So, nine months. I bet you had enough milk stored to last way beyond that."

"Sixteen months," she says with pride.

There isn't an upside to every story, but this deep freezer full of milk is Leigh's. It was a big price to pay and I tell her how amazing she was to persevere. Before parting, I give her my cell number and offer to help her stay ahead of any potential oversupply issue should she decide to breastfeed her second-born in her new city.

I believe she will be a better practitioner when caring for lactating mothers in her private practice. That, perhaps, is another upside.

Prime Time Live

A Sad Reason for 10 Minutes of Fame

*The health care system and its complex
relationship with the insurance industry
failed these families.*

What precipitated my brief minutes of fame was a cluster of tragedies. Once these cases were reported, the *Prime Time Live* crew, two camera men and a journalist taking Diane Sawyer's place, arrived at our hospital in 1998. The camera crew rounded with me in patient rooms, as I talked to mothers all afternoon. As we walked down the hall, I recall the men admiringly commenting to each other when they saw a framed certificate signed by Hugh Downs, on behalf of the U.S. committee for UNICEF, where he served as Chairman of the Board. (Ironically, Mr. Downs was from my hometown of Akron, Ohio.) The certificate he had signed affirmed our hospital's intent to seek the designation of a Baby-Friendly Hospital. The requirements for the designation assured that a hospital is complying with best-known practices to support breastfeeding. One of those practices includes assuring that breastfed babies have early, appropriate follow-up care. Dr. Ballard ordered two visits by home care nurses prior to the pediatrician visit. I attribute this decision to assuring our breastfed babies were protected.

Mothers held their babies close as we discussed how their breastfeeding experience was going and what to expect in the early days at home. Following this, the crew recorded an interview between the journalist and me.

Five babies, 5 to 14 days old (average 10 days old), had been admitted to the local Children's Hospital over a 5-month period for treatment for dehydration and other sequela. Ten percent is usually the upper acceptable limit of weight loss in the first days of life. The average weight loss for these babies upon readmission was 23 percent. It was frightening to hear each of their stories from their neonatal nutritionist. At that time, their hospital had no lactation department. The nutritionist and several of the doctors turned to me for insight into how these tragedies could have happened. With each call, the stories began to unfold with eerie similarity: older (age 28 to 38), first-time mothers, relatively short hospital stays (average for the four vaginal deliveries, 33 hours, for the one cesarean-section, 48 hours), no pediatric visit after discharge, infrequent breastfeeding, weak suck, and each mother, college-educated.

Without conducting in-depth, interviews myself, it was impossible to understand exactly what had gone wrong with each particular case. We agreed that the mothers had been through too much already to be interviewed. What I did know was that upon admission, no mother produced milk when she first pumped at the hospital. Was this because her mature milk, which normally arrives by day 3, had never come in? They each had reported some leaking. Or was it that the stress of her baby's readmission inhibited the release of the milk, or worse, had dried it up altogether? I'd had a mother once tell me that she only breastfed for 5 months because, upon seeing the baby's daddy shot to death, she subsequently never made a drop of milk. Stress is powerful.

As I watched the *Prime Time* segment a few weeks later, I wasn't surprised that only two of the five mothers consented to be interviewed. As one described watching her newborn *wither away* on the ambulance drive to the hospital, I thought of how unfair it is to expect a first-time parent to distinguish between a baby who sleeps because he has a full tummy, and one who sleeps because he's getting inadequate calories and milk. I thought of how tired moms are after delivery and how difficult it is to recall the myriad of instructions they are given during their postpartum stay. The interviewer didn't mention that each new mother had a short hospital stay. At the time of these births, a new dictate from health insurance companies mandated shorter stays, 24 hours for vaginal births. Many neonatologists felt this was a strong contributing factor to the tragedies. I had done my best to navigate the interview without in any way sounding like I blamed the parents. I did not. Four of the five had taken a prenatal breastfeeding class, mind you. They'd tried their best to prepare. In my estimation, it was a sad systems failure—short hospital stays coupled with delayed follow-up.

I was invited to meetings that senior Children's hospital physicians and administrators had with insurance officials from several companies. I was able to provide input on what would best serve the mothers of breastfed babies, both during their hospital stay and after discharge. It took nearly a year, but the meetings led to states requiring that insurance companies cover a hospital stay of up to 48 hours for a routine birth and 96 hours for a cesarean birth. This remains the law of the land. The Academy of Pediatrics (AAP) then revised its guideline for how soon a breastfed infant should be seen by a health care provider. When I had my children 40 years ago, babies were not seen until they were 2-weeks-old. Now, the AAP recommends that babies have a physician or nurse practitioner follow-up visit between day 3 and 5 of life.

None of these five women delivered at our hospital. Fortunately, we had a policy in place that made these types of tragedies less likely. The timing of the two home visits that were ordered contributed to this: one visit at 24 hours post-discharge, the other, 48 hours later. Additionally, in 1995, cut-backs had not yet occurred within the health department, and public health nurses were available to make many of these home visits.

After the *Prime Time* coverage, positive strides were made along the care-continuum, from prenatal to post-discharge, all over the U.S. One month later I received a letter from Dr. Ted Greiner, a Swedish professor of International Child Health, with his own speculations of why the U.S. health care system was failing to be a safety net for babies. He had great insight into best breastfeeding practices around the world, had studied at New York's Cornell University, and had conducted some of the most detailed studies of breastfeeding practices in West Africa. His PhD work in nutrition focused on breastfeeding in Yemen. Dr. Greiner's curriculum vita also includes work with the World Alliance for Breastfeeding Action, whose focus is to protect, promote, and support breastfeeding. I was hearing from an expert. He insisted that women should be better educated during their pregnancy and be allowed longer hospital stays. He was certain that if more U.S. hospitals followed the Ten Steps to Successful Breastfeeding, as outlined by the World Health Organization, then babies would be discharged with breastfeeding better established.

In the end, one baby's jaundice was so severe that it crossed into the brain, causing permanent neurologic damage. Two babies had grade III brain bleeds. The consequences of this, only time would tell. One of the babies suffered a stroke. The parents of the fourth baby, born in February, called on a snowy day to cancel a follow-up appointment at the delivering hospital. The father mentioned that his son's leg seemed *a little blue*. Days later, this infant's leg was amputated secondary to an iliac artery thrombosis. The final baby, despite severe weight loss and dehydration, had no apparent other maladies. There was no getting around the fact that this *Prime Time* segment created so much fear about breastfeeding that the breastfeeding initiation rates in the country dipped for several months. How could it not?

Twenty years later, though infrequent, there are still feeding tragedies. Babies need very close follow-up after discharge and parents need to know when to supplement breastfeeding without any overlay of external or internal pressure, save keeping their little one safe. We're allies to this end: all parents, all health care providers, the insurance industry, and all lactation consultants.

Chapter Eleven

LACTATION INTERNS

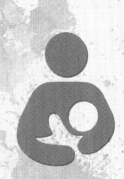

The First Lactation Intern Who Transformed a Near-Tragedy

In the midst of winter, I found there was within me, an invincible summer.

ALBERT CAMUS

Among the five mothers who endured the trauma of readmission of their newborn for dehydration, was a petite young woman from the east side of town. I met her five years after that event when she contacted me about providing her a 100-hour clinical internship in preparation to sit for the lactation board exam. I'd taken a course the summer of 1998 to learn to be a preceptor and decided to offer the program to Suzanne at no charge: a trial run, if you will.

Early in our meeting, she told me her story. Like the other newborns, he'd had significant weight loss, but unlike the others, there were no long-term negative consequences from this early event. Unlike the others, Suzanne made a successful transition to re-establishing both her supply and their breastfeeding relationship. She told me that she had trouble with latch in the hospital and went home with an appointment scheduled with the pediatrician for a 2-week check-up. As breastfeeding became more painful in the early days at home, she called into the pediatrician's office. "It's normal. Your nipples will eventually toughen up," she was mistakenly told by the woman taking calls that day. A few days after this, she called in again to report continued sore nipples, as well as constipation of her newborn. When the pediatrician heard about the constipation, he asked her to go straight to the emergency room. Breast milk has a laxative effect. A red flag had been raised.

A supportive pediatrician, as well as her own determination, helped turned things around for this couplet. Suzanne went on to join La Leche League, became a League leader, and one year after our internship, she became a board-certified lactation consultant. For these 18 years, she's used her experience to guide mothers in the early days and weeks of breastfeeding.

Training Pediatricians to Be Lactation Consultants

The things that you are passionate about are
not random, they are your calling.

FABIENNE FREDRICKSON

Over a 3-year period, I mentored two lactation interns who were attending pediatricians at our adjacent Children's Hospital. It was a period when the patient load was heavy and lactation staffing on the thin side. I think the strength of the program has always been the variety of cases we encounter at UCMC. As a tertiary care center, we have a plethora of unusual circumstances that surround many births, some of which are retold here. The diverse socioeconomic levels helped the young physicians see first-hand the impact of poverty on a mother's success with breastfeeding, from lack of support systems, to lack of transportation to get their milk to their premature, hospitalized infants. Everything is harder, except the act of breastfeeding itself, which creates a level playing field among the rich and poor, highly educated and minimally educated, and among the many races and cultures we serve at our hospital.

These physicians would eventually work for the Center for Breastfeeding Medicine, replacing Dr. Ballard upon her retirement. I was happy I could offer the internship to them. I hope it broadened their understanding of the enormous pressure delivering hospital staff is under to provide significant amounts of education, during a 36-hour stay that should have been received prenatally when the mothers aren't completely exhausted from giving birth. I hope it also helped them understand how mothers can go to them for follow-up, claiming never to have seen a lactation consultant during their stay. Postpartum can be a blur. Not to beat a dead horse, but this is why early follow-up of these babies is so crucial.

More on Lactation Interns

*The only person you are destined to become is
the person you decide to be.*

RALPH W. EMERSON

Besides physicians, over the years, lactation interns also included
a director of an infant and child development program in a nearby
county. Providing long-term follow up visits to young families, she
was in a pivotal position to influence both the duration of
breastfeeding and training of non-medical home visitors to be
supportive of their breastfeeding clients.

In 2011, I was happy to be a part of precepting a young
African American woman, because peer support can be so
influential in a young mother's life. This is also happening
more through personal and online breastfeeding support
groups like Mocha Moms, B.O.O.B.S. (Babies On Our Breasts),
and ROSE (Reaching Our Sisters Everywhere).

I asked this intern to go in with a resident to understand
why a mother was asking for formula. Once assured that the
request did not come from any latch pain, she facilitated the
discussion with the mother, noting that the baby's wets and
stools, feeding frequency, and weight were indicators of how
well her baby was, in fact, breastfeeding. The mother was
actively engaged in the discussion, sharing that not seeing
the milk just made her insecure. In addition, as one African
American mother to another, the LC intern addressed the

important, but delicate topic of the increased risk of sudden infant death among formula-fed infants, higher among the African American population. We are partners with *Cradle Cincinnati*, whose goal is that every child born in Hamilton County sees their first birthday. They remind us that "Nationally and locally, any fight for fewer infant deaths must begin with a fight for racial equity." The resident later told the LC it was the best education about breastfeeding she'd received all month. The balance of educating and helping a mom decide for herself isn't an easy task. I'm proud we're conveying ourselves in ways that empower the mom.

Chapter Twelve

THE NEWBORN INTENSIVE CARE

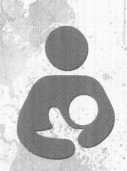

NICU Staff

*We all have the extraordinary coded
within us, waiting to be released.*

JL HOUSTON

Even over 25 years working as a lactation consultant, I wasn't able to intimately know the 87 nurses who serve in the NICU. There are just too many of them. You rub shoulders long enough, and care about them, you learn things that nudge you toward appreciation and compassion. There are so many things not said in a work setting—what a person is going through on any given day, neatly tucked in their locker at the beginning of the shift.

They arrive at 7 o'clock in the morning or evening, any evidence of hardship removed as they don their scrubs.

I listen to today's charge nurse. She's direct, some say confrontational, as she insists the physicians address a concern she feels has not received due focus. The residents learn not to take it personally, as they defend their position with research on any given topic. Sometimes they begin to understand a different perspective from the nurses, and they make adjustments to the plan of care today based on this charge nurse's prodding.

One nurse reminds me that her daughter is graduating from college this year and did I remember what happened after her birth. My memory is vague here. The baby transferred elsewhere a couple days after the birth. She revisits the story, filling in the details of how stressed she was, not being able to be the mom. Her nurse persona came out full force, and she was educating the other hospital's staff on the proper use of a new set of bilirubin lights, all the while appalled that she knew more than them. Mother Bear, the term she uses to describe herself.

Some of the nurses are quiet and it takes time to get to know them better. I assisted one nurse with breastfeeding her firstborn son, but the skin tag under his tongue so impeded tongue movement that his feedings always took an hour. While I pleaded with the attending nursery physician to evaluate this little boy's frenulum, he declined, simply saying he didn't *believe* in tongue-tie. She told me later that even bottle-feeding took an hour, and this was someone who could coax any hungry preemie to suck. She took the baby to an Ear, Nose, and Throat (ENT) specialist, who told her to just poke a bigger hole in the bottle. The nurse was incensed, and this soft-spoken woman found her voice, complaining to the doc that this was something one would tell someone in the hollers who had no access to modern-day medical care. Days before the director of ENT clipped the frenulum, her son had experienced choking, dusky-color episodes. Even for an experienced nurse, this was anxiety-provoking. Thank heavens the director agreed to the procedure, telling her that he clipped the frenulum of one of his own children. Her son is now in college, a long-distance runner who prides himself in running backwards at lighting speed. After she first delivered him, the nurse's mother visited and told me her own birth story, delivering my colleague in Venezuela, where her husband was working for a U.S. company. My friend was 10 weeks premature and discharged at a little over 3 pounds. Her mother was told to give bottles all but twice a day, but thinking that the country was backwards, she breastfed exclusively. My friend rolls her eyes and shakes her head, as if to say, from her lips to your ears.

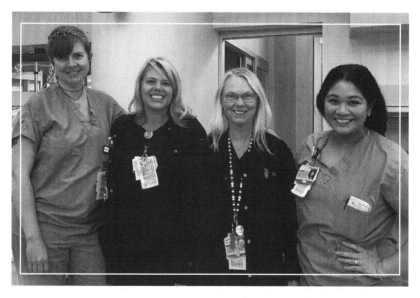

∗ 4 of 87 NICU nurses: Meaghan (CLC too), Laura, Becky, Gazen (currently nursing) ∗

Interspersed in my years there were celebrations of engagement, marriage, adoption, pregnancy, birth, and birth of grandchildren, as well as casseroles for the sick, heart-wrenching funerals for family members, summer outings at Barb's lake, Christmas parties at Mary's house, as well as job-change and retirement luncheons. And of course, in the midst of it, many babies saved and some babies lost, including some of their own. Through it all, they showed up and worked –7 a.m. to 7 p.m.

Certain staff, more than others, are gung-ho breastfeeding supporters. Many nurses have personal success stories, breastfeeding their own, from months to 3 years. A few have breastfed twins. Some weren't able to establish breastfeeding but did pump their milk, either loving it or hating it. A few, for all the effort to make it work, never established a supply, and yet remain committed to supporting the mothers in the unit. I take my hat off to them. I have a special admiration for a few nurses who were diagnosed and treated for breast cancer in their 30s, returning to work with a head wrap or an OR scrub cap, atop their heads.

Most nurses, though, have only breastfed full-term infants and at times are overly optimistic about how well a preemie has breastfed, and thus don't offer any additional supplement through the gavage tube that leads to the stomach. If the baby falls asleep after the feeding, this is proof enough for them. It took time before they would consider that a preemie that falls asleep may be tired after the feeding, not necessarily full. It took a scale accurate within half a teaspoon for them to see the amount of milk truly transferred. Even then, there is a skill to accurately weighing a baby before and after a breastfeeding session, and I suppose even I couldn't convince the skeptics who'd had one too many babies register a negative number, as though in that 15 minutes they'd lost weight instead of gained.

I especially admire nurses for whom breastfeeding wasn't easy or successful. Still, they persist as enthusiastic advocates to the young moms. One such nurse had breastfed two children for 6 months. Immediately after the delivery of her third, her husband noted a lump a few inches below her left collar bone. Over the coming 4 weeks it increased in size and tenderness. She was sent for an ultrasound, which yielded inconclusive results. This was followed by a biopsy 2 weeks later—an unusual choice for a lactating woman. The long needle was inserted several times to obtain tissue from different parts of the area, then a titanium chip was inserted at the site so that if there was ever a question about the lump in the future, it would be identified as previously examined and benign. This was followed by a few sutures to close the incision. It was at this point that I saw her in the NICU and learned of her ordeal. She described the procedure as painful and burning. Throughout it all, she'd heroically continued to breastfeed. She asked if I would examine her in one of the NICU pump rooms. It looked angry, bright red, and was tender to touch. It seemed likely to be infected tissue. I suggested she have one of UCMC's breast specialists examine it. The physician diagnosed a fistula, caused by a punctured milk duct during the biopsy. Milk was now accumulating in the tissue with nowhere to exit. She was prescribed an antibiotic, but before the medicine kicked in, the fistula ruptured through her skin and milk and pus oozed down her belly.

Still, she continued breastfeeding. At intermittent times during the day, she gently massaged the fistula to empty the milk through her skin. Several weeks later, it had completely healed. Each time we saw one another at work, I received an update.

"How did you ever continue on with breastfeeding while enduring all this?

"I was committed," she replied with a confident smile. Ironically, she nursed this baby a year, twice as long as the first two. You bond with staff in the telling of stories, no matter the topic, but especially when it's about breastfeeding dilemmas. I certainly would have understood if she'd weaned instead of opting to persevere.

Some staff never realized they signed-on for assisting with breastfeeding when they applied for a job with critical premature infants. As one nurse said, "I don't do breasts." However, most step up to the plate. It's likely awkward, especially if they've not breastfed or had their own children. But practice with assisting mothers can build confidence and help nurses feel more at ease. It just takes a willingness to make that first step. One nurse did so with a tad bit of inconsistency. Going through a pod once, she realized I'd overheard her say she didn't like to help with breastfeeding, and flung her hand over her mouth in embarrassment.

"It's just weird," she explained. I stopped to talk about it briefly. Some don't like to hold babies during spinal-tap procedures, but they do what's called for. I hope our discussion gave the nurse the latitude to name her feelings. I reminded her that moms really appreciate it when she sets her feelings aside and rolls up her sleeves to help. While she's not a stellar breastfeeding advocate, she's risen to the occasion. I see that her particular cutting edge of growth is to be proactive in her support, not waiting for mothers to ask if they can breastfeed.

You don't change attitudes or practices by criticizing people. Nurses need to feel they can share honestly. And you can't change what you don't admit. I'd rather have a staff member express her ambivalence or discomfort with the breastfeeding process without judgment because being heard and accepted softens attitudes. People are generally receptive toward me, perhaps in part, because of this.

About 72 percent of the mothers with babies in our NICU pump milk for their babies. Most want to directly breastfeed. It's a busy unit with nurses caring for sicker babies alongside more stable babies who are ready to breastfeed. The nurses have their work cut out for them. I feel extremely fortunate to have been part of the team. They are committed to saving lives. If you've ever had a critically ill child, you know the kind of gratitude one holds for those who helped your child heal. It's a gratitude that lasts a lifetime.

The Quadruplets and My Dad

He would walk into my mind as if it were
a town and he a torchlight procession of one,
lighting up the streets.

UNKNOWN

In December of 1995, a consult was ordered for a mother, pregnant with quadruplets, who was restricted to bedrest on the High-Risk OB unit. Meeting Lisa that day was the beginning of a 20-month relationship that culminated two years later when I published my first paper in a scientific journal.

Professional papers report findings of potential import to other health care providers caring for similar patients. With only one other study about quads and breastfeeding up to that date, my hope was to broaden the understanding of how best to support the breastfeeding process for higher order (i.e., greater than twins) multiples. Case reports like this aren't generalizable to all, but they open a window of insight into an experience shared by a small minority of women. In 2013, a Center for Disease Control (CDC) report on higher order births indicated that only 270 sets were born in the U.S. that year. This represents .00007% of the year's 3.9 million births.

I co-authored this paper with Karen Kerkoff-Gromada, author of *Mothering Multiples*. What a professional paper doesn't allow us to include is the backstory. I found this story equally compelling. Lisa was then a 34-year-old married mother with a 9-year-old, conceived naturally. Many pregnancy attempts and years later, she saw a fertility expert and was successfully carrying four babies. She spoke to me with pride about her success with breastfeeding her son, Kyle, who nursed for 2-and-a-half years. She hoped to do the same with these babies, an ambitious undertaking even for a singleton birth. I was fascinated while listening to her determined attitude, and I asked her if I might follow her and the babies through this experience and report the outcomes in a medical journal. She was happy to comply.

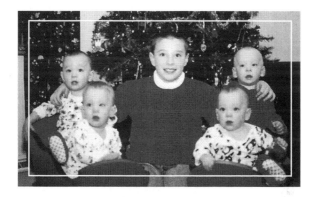

＊ *The quadruplets and big brother then...* ＊

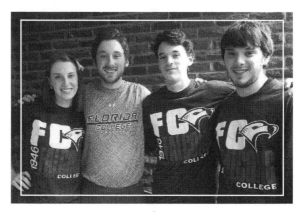

＊ *... and now* ＊

Your professional life doesn't proceed in a vacuum. It's surrounded by the *rest* of your life, with its various joys, heartbreaks, peaks, and mundane periods. I was not able to be there at the birth because it happened the same day I was called out-of-town to my hospitalized father's bedside. Returning to work was necessary, but not easy. The quads were 2-days-old at that time. My dad passed away 22 days after their birth, and that date is forever intertwined with Lisa and her babies. I think dad needed, not one, but four little angels to replace him on this earth.

Born 9 weeks early, Katie, Justin, Eric, and Connor, had a fairly stable hospital course. Lisa was busy pumping within 2 hours of their birth. Once she was discharged, it was hard to keep up with the recommended 12 pumping sessions per 24 hours, but she was doing the best she could. It was going to take time to rebuild her strength after the muscle loss from her 11-week course of bedrest. Lisa's supply was stubbornly stuck at a volume enough for only two babies. When they were 11 days old, I suggested she get a thyroid level drawn. It was a full year before she followed through and discovered that her thyroid was, at least in part, a contributor to her low supply. (Though, can you call a supply great enough for twins "low"?) It's always an illuminating moment when you begin to question what makes a person follow or postpone following your professional advice. The experience was a foreshadowing for what I would later term, *maternal pacing*. In short, mothers do what they can at the pace that is achievable for them.

Can anyone make enough for quadruplets anyway? The answer is yes, and Lisa had firsthand experience here. She developed a friendship with another quads mom who delivered at a nearby hospital a month after her. This mom had no intention of direct breastfeeding, but was easily making enough for four babies. We know from the literature, European wet nurses fed upwards of 17 children simultaneously. Lisa was calm and easy-going, and this news from her friend proved no deterrent to her commitment to pump. She taught me a lot about accepting what is and making the most of it.

I don't think you have quads and get organized. I think organization must be in your DNA if you're even open to considering managing multiples; at least it was for Lisa. Her babies had staggered discharges after 3-to-5-week hospital stays. Prior to that, she was offering each one of them the breast at the hospital. She never attempted breastfeeding simultaneously, but it was her intent to do this once they became more proficient nursers at home.

When I began regular home visits, I saw her day's schedule was a well-oiled machine. Her husband, Wade, worked evening shift, and her parents came over every night of the first year without fail. They helped feed, get babies to sleep, and made sure Kyle got plenty of attention as well. Eventually, Lisa returned to work part-time cleaning at her church. She added this systematically into their schedule and life went on.

Her pattern was to rotate breastfeeding two babies per feeding, occasionally pump, and tend to the routine household chores a parent shares with their spouse. And while I had lots of clever ideas about how to facilitate breastfeeding, Lisa didn't really need me. Frankly, once I was in her home environment, it was easy to see why some of my suggestions were unrealistic. She did what worked for her and the babies. This was part of my own take home message from the experience.

It wasn't how much Lisa breastfed that mattered to her; it was that she wanted to offer the breast for the same *amount of time* as she'd done with Kyle. This was her personal goal. And indeed, Justin, Katie, and Eric breastfed for 2 and a half years, and Connor weaned at 11 months.

Don't underestimate *maternal pacing*. I think it's key to helping moms reach achievable goals. We, as health care professionals, discover it, not by dictating what *should* be done, but by helping a mom name what *can* be done in the scheme of what's best for them and their babies. I am not always successful at being an attentive listener, but when I can validate mom's concerns, get to the bottom of misperceptions, and empathize—that's when moms seem most empowered to discover their own solutions. Just as preemies need their feedings paced, so the milk doesn't overwhelm them and cause them to stop breathing, so too, mothers pace themselves. I think we do mothers a service when we respect the pace and manner in which each woman assumes her role as mother. That outcome will always be best, even when it's not the one we expected.

The Alcoholic and
Her Twin Preemies

*I admit to more caution when it comes to drinking,
even aside from breastfeeding. I think we have a huge,
condoned problem in this country. My standard guide
is that there's no reason for a breastfeeding mother
to have more than one or two small drinks on a given
day, once or twice in a given week; and this preferably
after nursing.*

She is pumping a huge supply of milk for her barely-three-pound twins in the NICU, when I hear from a nurse that dad asked about the appropriateness of drinking while pumping. I'm paged after he's brought it up to a third nurse, asking, "So it's okay that she's drinking and pumping?"

I go back and poured over her prenatal paper chart. And there it is, intermittent participation in a 12-step program with little drinking in the pregnancy, and two DUIs prior to the pregnancy. I wonder who's defining *little* and how. This latter information tells me she may be forthright with her doctor because she didn't have to acknowledge the DUIs during the history-taking. She must be off the wagon.

Although alcohol moves in and out of mother's milk in much the same way it does out of the blood stream, it's risky business to counsel moderation with a habitual user. In fact, I am appalled when I see Facebook posts, however well intended, about the benign nature of drinking and breastfeeding, as though this information sent out blindly and reposted God knows where, suffices for good counsel. When I'm with a mother for months in the NICU, know her social behavior, and she asks if it's all right to have a glass of wine for her birthday, I'm not hesitant to say yes. The difference is—I know the mother I'm counseling.

I see so many problems with this mom's scenario. Will she be too impaired to care for the twins once they're home, too impaired to drive (or remember that she shouldn't drive) if there were an emergency? No amount of pumping and dumping will make up for poor judgement if she falls asleep with one of them in a chair. Then there are the babies. Breastfed babies tend to eat less in the 24 hours after a mother's moderate drinking. And if she's drinking heavily, say, every other day, failure to thrive could be on the horizon. Then there's the fact that foods flavor breastmilk. I wouldn't want those twins "preferring" beer in their adolescence. The acceptability of heavy drinking in this country is staggering. We don't need to tip the scales toward it for the next generation.

We chat at the bedside in Pod A, her steel grey eyes dance as she presses her lips against the forehead of her son. Regine is an affable 25-year-old mother, wearing white dress slacks and a nice navy blue blouse. Her hair and make-up are in place. I sit close to her holding her other daughter as together we reflect on the question daddy posed to the staff. She doesn't show the least bit of annoyance over his disclosure, acknowledging she knows he has her and the kids' best interest at heart. "I just needed to know the rules about drinking and breastmilk, that's all," she explains, not grasping the broader concern for her well-being (and the babies' after discharge). She's aware that we can test her milk randomly during her babies' hospitalization. Before leaving that day, she meets privately with our social worker, talking in more detail than is in my jurisdiction to discuss. She went back to AA meetings, and weeks later, the twins are discharged home to dad and her, along with a cooler of her plentiful supply of frozen milk.

The Porcelain Pacifier, Symbol of Regret

When challenge is present,
the teacher is in the room.

UNKNOWN

Dr. Ballard and I have been asked by the OB medical director to consult with one of his patients, pregnant and in her mid-third trimester. She is a 52-year-old physician from a nearby city, pregnant via in vitro fertilization. She is only 8 years younger than Dr. Ballard (Jeanne), who will be retiring from neonatology in a short 6 years. We meet in the lactation department office after her separate meeting with Jeanne. This patient reminds me so much of Mrs. Lutz, my third-grade teacher, both in appearance and mannerisms. She is sweetness to the core, and pleasant yet reserved. I take a liking to her immediately.

She and her husband are hoping to avoid a C-section. We talk about greeting her son with a long period of skin-to-skin holding, reviewing the benefits of maintaining his body temperature, stabilizing his heart and respiratory rate, hardwiring his brain, and bonding–of course, bonding. She seems mesmerized by it all, smiling and sighing. She tells me that even if she ends up having a C-section, she doesn't want to miss out on this bonding experience in that first hour. We discuss the basics of exclusive breastfeeding while viewing a PowerPoint I'd updated the prior year. She has a good idea of what to expect in those early days by the time we finish, but I forward the lecture to her for later review. As a professional courtesy, I give her my pager number should she want to talk again.

Less than three weeks later, she contacts me to let me know she'll be having a C-section after all, and asks if I wouldn't mind attending the delivery. I let her know I've never done this before, usually meeting moms in the Recovery Room (RR), but I promise to check with her doctor and the nurse-manager of Labor and Delivery. With their approval, I come in early the following Thursday, don a gown, and scrub in. She's 34 weeks along, so the baby will be considered late preterm and will be watched closely to assure he transitions well to life outside the womb, while making sure he maintains his body temperature and eats. Any of these three activities can be a bump in the road for a baby born this early.

When I enter the OR, the baby and placenta are delivered. Dad is holding the swaddled newborn near mom in her eye's view. They are over-the-moon thrilled. We're 20 minutes in, and I ask if the circulating nurse has taken the baby's vitals. When she says she hasn't, I offer to do it for her. I lay their son briefly on the pram under the warmer so that I can observe him, watching his chest and counting his breathes. Tyler is stable; a little bubbly at his lips, but this isn't unusual. He has mild flaring of his nostrils, something to keep an eye on, but his chest rises and falls with ease. I swaddle him again and as he lay in my arms, I begin to listen to his heart rate with a stethoscope. As I count, across the room, I see the attending neonatologist come in the door. He has paused NICU rounds, to check on this baby. He speaks briefly to the OB. Our eyes meet; he mouths "OK?" I nod, and he returns to his rounds in the NICU. As I hand Tyler back to dad, he grunts a wet cough, then settles. Dad looks to me for reassurance.

Mom is ready to be wheeled to RR, but wants to get her baby to her chest. The staff led the discussion toward waiting yet another 2 minutes until she is in the RR. As expected, she accommodates. One day, one day, I think, babies will be against their mom's body while they are still being sewn up, but not today. In moments, they are skin to skin. She is in bliss. Tyler isn't showing cues to breastfeed yet. Being 6 weeks early, we give him some help by sliding his body close enough that he can whiff the scent of her breast. He nests there comfortably, except for a few grunts that make me uneasy. I observe with vigilance. She tickles his lip with her nipple, but he's unresponsive, save another couple grunts. He doesn't seem as pink to me, and I turn to the RR nurse who is responsible for transporting babies to the NICU when needed. She sees the caution in my eyes and nods in agreement that Tyler should be transported to the NICU, but she is just about to get mom's blood pressure. I offer to transport him, not thinking much about it, since I was once a Pediatric ICU nurse myself.

As I wheel Tyler, the less than 3-minute ride to the NICU, dad returns to the OR where he'd just realized he'd left his camera. The baby seems paler as we fly through the halls, and in the small space of skin visible above the blanket near his neck, I can see his chest retracting, telling me it's taking him more effort to breathe. As I enter the NICU, I call to the attending doctor, and he points me to the Pod adjacent to where he's gathered with the residents. Margaret, assigned as Tyler's nurse, receives him in Pod B, attaches a pulse oximeter to interpret how well his blood is oxygenated, and grabs the O2 tubing to provide blow-by oxygen. We would expect his oxygen saturation to be above 90%, but it's 77%, and slow to rise as oxygen is provided.

I feel sick. I should have turned on oxygen as we were wheeling to the NICU and could kick myself for this omission, as well as for not letting the RR nurse transport the baby.

I'm the lactation consultant. It's not my job to transport babies. But we are past that now. Margaret is calling for the assistance of the neonatal fellow and the respiratory therapist. I am reeling with anxiety and feel too upset to stay in the unit, in fact, I feel too upset to even see my assigned patients on the Mother-Baby unit. I pass the father in the hallway and he asks how to get to the NICU. Normally, I'd walk a parent to the unit myself. I can't. I'm too stressed and I'm sure he sees it in my eyes and now he too has a worried look on his face.

I leave the hospital and arrive home in 10 minutes. Immediately, I page the mother's physician, our medical director. His reassurances don't calm me. "Quit flagellating yourself. He's 34 weeks. I knew he'd have RDS." Respiratory Distress Syndrome, in this case, is caused by lungs that are immature and deficient in surfactant, a lipid/protein complex substrate that reduces surface tension and prevents collapse of the lung's alveolar sacs when the baby exhales. It would be rare for a 35-week baby to be deficient, but this is a 34-weeker and the more preterm a baby is, the more likely he will have RDS. Still, I feel no consolation.

By early afternoon, I page Ed, the neonatologist on-call. He tells me the baby is stable but guarded. I assure him that when I obtained the respiratory rate, the baby was on the pram and I was actually looking at his chest. Tyler wasn't in my arms, as he may have presumed. He understands. They have intubated the baby and the ventilator provides a means of giving synthetic surfactant.

I wonder if I will live with this anxiety the next 3-and-a half weeks of the baby's stay. By 2 weeks, he is off all breathing support, save oxygen via nasal cannula. Mom's supply is above his need, not stellar, but adequate. She begins to offer the breast once he is ready to feed by mouth. He is slow to progress but it's important that we give her adequate time for breastfeeding attempts. I've studied 181 babies who breastfed before they started bottle-feeding, and we learned they are nearly four times as likely to go home breastfeeding if they've been afforded this opportunity.

As I help her, I coo and smile and make note of his unique cuteness, but inside, my heart is always racing. Mom is pleased with the progress, however faltering. Dr. Ballard stops by a few times and gives encouragement as mom and I work together, and she tries her hand at assisting with latching the baby on as well.

During one of our latch appointments, mom makes a point to tell me, given the fact that he was going to go to the NICU, she wouldn't have traded those 20 minutes in Recovery Room, holding her son skin to skin, for the world. I'm glad she feels that way. I just don't share the feeling.

By discharge, Tyler is better at bottle-feeding, that is, it takes him less time and he takes in more milk. Mom is there to breastfeed twice a day, and the other six feedings, he is offered a bottle, including once a day when dad feeds. Tyler has more practice bottle-feeding, so it's no surprise. Still, I'm disappointed because I so want everything to proceed perfectly for this couplet.

On our last day together, she gives Jeanne and me gifts she's bought at a fine jewelry store in her hometown—hers, a guardian

angel looking over an infant, mine a porcelain pacifier. We thank
her and say goodbye. Jeanne has given the mom her personal
cell, and she calls several times for advice and undoubtedly,
encouragement. She has no idea how relieved I am that she's
calling Jeanne and not me. I just want to put the whole experience
behind me, but that will take many, many months.

As the memory is finally fading, Margaret, Tyler's admitting
nurse approaches me. It's a good 8 months later. She wants me
to sign-off on a document for her clinical ladder merit advancement
form. She tells me it's about helping transition Tyler from a 77%
pulse oxygen rate to well above 90%. It all comes back to me in
a rush. I can't even bring myself to read her documentation. She's
an excellent nurse. I've no doubt that it's thorough, and I go
against protocol and sign without ever having read it.

Once restless nights fade to sound sleep, I am left with only
one memento—her gratitude expressed in a porcelain pacifier.
It sits year after year in the back of my china cabinet. Though
it should remind me of a good outcome, it only prompts regret.

The Triplets' Dad

Our first experience of life is primarily felt in the body. Our mother's gaze is our first relational imprinting. Her early mirroring stays with us our whole lives. I am sure you have seen how mother and child fix on each other with total delight during breastfeeding. It is almost eucharistic. We know ourselves in the security of those who love us and gaze upon us.

RICHARD ROHR

OFM

Christmas photos came for three or four years after the triplets' discharge. I recall this family of five so vividly, in part, because I'd never had a dad so committed to holding his babies skin to skin, this six-foot, lanky optometrist. He and mom rotated babies like hot dogs on a campfire spit, always keeping one or two of them close during their lengthy visits. Screens around him? Nope, he didn't care. No breasts, after all. And holding his babies more in the open, he could engage the staff with ease and show off those tiny babies.

He read everything he could get his hands on about this method of holding, often referred to as Kangaroo Care. Now there is a plethora of literature in lay and scientific journals about this way of being an active participant in a baby's growth and health. Tim often referred to feeling most like their father when he held them against his chest. It's a powerful protective symbol, beyond the nurturing symbol often accorded it.

Yes to keeping their babies warm, yes to stabilizing their heart and respiratory rates, yes to bonding, yes to warmth, yes to better blood sugars, but equally valuable, Tim and Valerie were providing low tech brain-building as they held their little ones skin to skin, reclining in chairs or sitting in rockers for long periods.

This activity is another great economic leveler. You don't have to have money, or for that matter, be a breastfeeder; you simply need to take off your shirt and relax. Neurons are forming; hard-wiring of the brain is happening at exponential rates during skin-to-skin contact. I learn through a *DandleLion* webinar that at birth, a baby's brain is made up of about one hundred billion neurons, roughly the same number of stars in the Milky Way. Indeed, these children will know that security because of the loving gaze of both mother and father.

A few months after discharge, Valerie wrote to say breastfeeding was continuing to go well for all three, and that their family was moving to Florida where her parents lived, and she added, "...where there will be two more chests for our babies."

The Bubblegum Thief

When Patients Rob You of Trust

---

*I keep my ideals because, in spite of everything, I
still believe that people are really good at heart.*

ANNE FRANK

In September 2004, two weeks before my daughter's wedding, I
had to work well into the evening. Before leaving, I swing by the
NICU to drop off paperwork, and see a mother sitting on the staff
side of the clerk's desk. Peculiar site, this uncommon occurrence,
even more so because she's in her PJs. I knew she'd been discharged
two days prior. Parents often spend the night when their baby is
being discharged the following day, or when their baby is critical.
But neither of these were part of the equation.

"What's up?" I ask, as she looks down despondently at the
phone on the desk.

"I can't find a ride home and I've already been here 6 hours."

"Hm, where do you live, Cierra?"

"Near Tri-county mall," she replies, as she looks up at me
so innocently.

This is only 10 to 15 minutes out of my way, so I offer her
a ride. Grateful, she gathers her supplies, gives her daughter
a farewell pat, and joins me at the elevator. Cierra's easy to
engage and tells me why she's in pajamas.

"Basically, I just didn't bother to get dressed today," she admits.

If I'd heard this from another mom, a red flag may be waving concerning postpartum depression, but nothing about her mannerisms suggest this. As we get into the car, I toss my purse in the backseat. Recalling her long visit, I assume she may be hungry, and remove my bulky, yellow wallet, setting it between us. A fast food restaurant is blocks away. We exit the employee parking garage and I notice a white plastic grocery bag on the floor. "Is that your breast pump tubing," I ask, with a nod in its direction? Cierra's is doing well with a pumping schedule, but even one 6-to-8-hour gap can precipitate a decrease in her supply.

"No, it's my dishes. I brought in my dinner."

On hearing this, I both worry about her supply and silently admire her forethought to bring in food. Exiting the garage, I turn left down the road, away from the restaurant. We chat about her supply, other children, but mostly we talk about current events. The Bush versus Kerry campaign is in full swing, and coming into home stretch. She acknowledges that, at 26, this will be her first time to vote. She speaks with aplomb about issues, particularly those that affect her: jobs, the cost of groceries, the limits and cost of public transportation. It isn't me, but Cierra, who brings up the lack of weapons of mass destruction and the Iraq War. I'm kind of amazed. The drive passes quickly, and I drop her off in the parking lot of a large apartment complex, near Costco and Target. It's roughly 10:30.

Arriving home, I gather my purse from the back seat and remember my wallet. It's not on the seat. Perhaps it dropped to the floor or under the seat. I'm perplexed. Thinking I'm overlooking it, I ask my 18-year-old son to search with a flashlight. He comes up empty-handed. "That's weird," I say aloud to him. Could it have fallen out in her parking lot? Surely, she didn't take it, with its checks, cash, mementos—two weeks before my daughter's wedding. I call into the NICU and ask the clerk for mom's number. I can only recall the first three digits of the exchange and the one she's reading me doesn't match. Crap.

Now I'm driving 30 minutes back to the unit to retrieve her record in my locked office. As I walk into the NICU, the clerk advises me to file a police report, as she's been on the Internet and sees that mom has a prior record of theft. She hands me a paper with the address and phone number of the police department in the mother's district.

I dial, begin to tell my story, but mid-sentence, am interrupted by the officer who says that this isn't something handled over the phone. I have to go in. It's 11:30 by the time I leave the hospital. The shortest route to the station takes me through a county park just two blocks from home. I travel it daily. And while I know that a ticket on this stretch of deserted road would be pricy, I speed along, eager to file the report as soon as possible. About midnight, I am pulled over by flashing lights. I tell the officer why I'm speeding, as he's retrieving his pad and pen and asking for my license. Inauthentic tears are bubbling at the corners of my eyes. He seems unmoved by my story, but I think to tell him that I spoke to an officer at the station just 40 minutes prior. This gets his attention. He excuses himself and returns to his squad car to verify my story. Back to my car five minutes later, he warns me, regardless of circumstances and time of day, I cannot drive 50 in a 25 mph zone. Did I know the cost of the ticket he wasn't giving me? Of course not. Did I know that fines double on federal roads? Thank God, I'd mistakenly called the police station from the hospital so that someone could corroborate my story.

I roll into the station another ten minutes later and repeat the story to the officer at the desk. "By the way," he asks, "what's her name?" As I say it, his eyes widen. He reaches across his desk and pulls the top file in a large stack. "I've been looking for her forever."

He finishes his report, thanks me, and says he'll be in touch. As I walk out the door, in what seemed like an afterthought, he recommends I contact my credit card companies. It's dawning on me that this has ramifications beyond the cash and sentimentals in the wallet, but I feel confident that I'm ahead of the game. After all, earlier she'd tried to get a ride home, to no avail. What's the likelihood, she'd be out and about at 12:30? Still, as remote as it might be, I held out a small hope that the wallet was simply on the pavement where I'd dropped her off.

I'm back home shortly after one a.m., and tell my son the story as he shakes his head in disbelief.

"You'd better call Visa before you wake dad," he prods.

When I reach customer service, the woman on the other end of the line is almost chuckling as I speak.

"Honey, we shut that down a good hour ago. We figured that card was either stolen or you were in some sort of manic shopping frenzy!" It's amazing this could be detected so quickly, but good grief, what has this mama done? "Well," she continues, "first she went to the gas station, and then she went shopping at Biggs. Looks like once she finished shopping, her driver went in and shopped as well."

"Are we talking a couple hundred dollars?" I ask, incredulous.

"Try a couple thousand, $1,816.52 to be exact." I am stunned as I consider both the blatant betrayal and the wedding expenses that were now rolling in.

Two days later, I receive a call from the officer. He and a partner had gone to the apartment after we'd parted. There were still many unpacked bags of merchandise when they arrived. The refrigerator was full. This last piece of news tugs at my heartstrings. No one in America should be going hungry. He continues that, without a warrant, they searched the apartment with her cooperation. Under the bed, they found her boyfriend, who'd just been released from jail that day. He wasn't involved in Cierra's crime, and didn't want to be arrested again. He wasn't. She ratted out the neighbor who couldn't pick her up from the hospital at 8, but was free to take her shopping at 11. The police gathered the non-perishable merchandise from both apartments.

Meanwhile, at the hospital, within days, we are out of Cierra's frozen milk and have to switch the baby to formula. For me, the wedding is fast approaching, and I am without a credit card.

I hadn't heard a thing for a week, when the clerk of a county judge phones me on my cell. The judge would like me to recommend a consequence for the mother. I feel much ambivalence about being pulled into her life in this way, but he assures me the burden was not mine. The final decision rests solely with the judge. Grandma has custody of the other two kids, so I know that jail time would not be a hardship for them. Ultimately, I said I think children learn what they live, and at least she should be required to participate in parenting classes.

"Jail time?" he asks. The question lingers.

I know she's had a prior arrest for theft, yet it didn't seem the prior conviction with jail time created a deterrent for her future actions. This should be the judge's determination. I silently begin to consider the ramifications. How would this effect future employment? What negative influences would surround Cierra in jail? In the end, I don't know what was decided. The staff said that after a few weeks, she was coming to see the baby in the evenings. Perhaps she is avoiding me. Perhaps this is the only time she can get a ride.

On the day of the baby's discharge, I am in a conference room when a colleague walks in with Cierra. "I think you owe Chris an apology, don't you?" she says emphatically. Clearly, Cierra is caught off guard. Together they sit down across from me. She is quick to say she didn't steal the wallet. It had "gotten stuck to her grocery bag by bubble gum." I could barely contain a laugh.

But the nurse is having none of this and says, "I can tell you that's a ridiculous excuse. But even if it were true, you went shopping, for God sake."

"Well, I have to give you that," she replies calmly. The nurse went on a few minutes about betraying the trust of someone who was offering an act of kindness. The two of us sit in awkward silence before I decide to get up and leave.

Later, the nurse mentions that she'd advised the mom to write me a note of apology before leaving with her baby. It never happened. For a few days, it made the rounds among the 87 NICU nurses, the docs, and social worker, and I was duly chided. Several weeks after my daughter's wedding, the topic is finally off the table. No one is teasing me anymore.

It's three years later now and I walk into the Mother-Baby unit. A bubbly woman rushes up to me with an affectionate greeting. To be honest, by that time, I didn't recall her face, but when she said "Cierra," it registers. By this interchange, no one would guess the way our paths converged in September of 2004. You may have thought us friends. And who's to say we weren't? She had the same pleasant disposition I'd found endearing before. Standing in the hall, Cierra goes on about how her near 3-year-old is doing, and how she moved an hour away and is getting her life together. The baby, born the day prior, is full-term, going home with mom, and exclusively breastfeeding.

The Lawyer and Her Morning Beer

Ninety percent of life is just showing up.

WOODY ALLEN

During my work in the NICU, I'd secured a grant to be able to provide a Lunch and Learn on a monthly basis for the pumping moms. These gatherings were often lively, sometimes sobering, but always supportive for the mothers.

A well-dressed, though slightly disheveled mother, bustles into the conference room 10 minutes late, apologizes as she sits down with the rest of the moms. She doesn't even pause to get the drift of where the group discussion is, but blurts out that she'd had an awkward conversation with her father-in-law that morning. He'd come to pick her up to drive her to the hospital to see her premature son. Without knocking, he'd walked around to the back of the house and entered directly into the kitchen. There was the mother of his first grandchild, sipping a beer at 9 a.m., laptop in front of her.

"Julia, do you want to talk about what's going on?" he asks. She'd no idea what his question or tone of voice referred to. With a pregnant pause between them, he finally points to what was so obviously wrong with the picture.

"Oh my gosh, you're worried I'm drinking?" She invites him to sit down, and she bends over in laughter at this retelling.

She proceeds to explain that she'd been on the Internet searching for how to increase her milk supply. She was only making about half of what her baby required. Several articles in the lay literature indicated that beer is a common supply-booster. When she asked a few neighbors what they thought, one of them nodded in agreement. "My German grandmother swore by it."

I don't know if her German grandmother swore by beer because, after all, she's German, or if she thought it helped her supply. There is disputed evidence that the hops in beer, a good source of vitamin B6, may enhance supply, but it would be better to take a small amount of B6, than to start drinking a daily beer. And B6 in too high a quantity can decrease a supply. I had to admit that our European neonatologist had recently told me that they developed non-alcoholic beer in Switzerland specifically for the lactating mother, though I think that was just for drinking, not supply-boosting. While he wanted me to add it to a handout titled, *Tips to Increase Milk Supply*, I cautiously declined.

There are several other non-alcoholic options available for supply-building that are utilized around the world. I offer the mother and the group this explanation and the other options. I'm sure her father-in-law will thank me.

The Grandfather Who Donated Goat's Milk

The only gift is a portion of thyself. The poet gives his poem, the painter, his picture; the shepherd, his lamb.

RALPH WALDO EMERSON

SELF-RELIANCE

She has delivered preterm twins, tiny enough that their care providers will want to protect these small babies' guts from the foreign protein of another mammal. This is not her first birth, and past experience tells her she'll have plenty of milk. But this level of prematurity means mom will be totally dependent on an electric pump and her hands to express milk, and this isn't just one baby, it's two. The docs say she's declined to consent to donor milk from the certified milk bank, despite the fact it's sterile and millions of ounces have been utilized for preemies, with no adverse effects. They ask me to see her, give a more in-depth explanation, and answer any lingering questions.

She's just finishing her second pump session when I arrive, and she's perplexed that she's only eking out drops—drip, drip, drip, like the milk at the bottom of a carton, only you can't take this container and shake it upside down. The first session yielded just over an ounce, and she's confused about why she would make less milk than the first time. Worried, she's beginning to rethink the donor milk and asks for more information before I even offer it.

She nods with genuine interest during my 5-minute spiel, but afterward, the conversation takes an unexpected turn. She asks if we could give her babies goat's milk instead, explaining how she vividly recalls her grandpa, a rural farmer, helping sick babies by donating some of his goats' milk to the country doctor who resided down the road. With a simple explanation, she understood it wasn't the cow specifically that was the problem; it was, instead, the non-human mammal, despite the fact that a goat's protein is less allergenic. It wasn't a farfetched idea. I tell her that in Namibia, a mother with a low supply does use goat's milk for her healthy term infant.

In the end, she declined the pasteurized donor milk, a rarity at our hospital. It turned out not to matter. Her supply rose rapidly and she made enough for triplets. Her twins consumed only her milk.

The Japanese Grandmother

A Collison Course of Culture and Science

*Many cultures like Japan, cement this
natural bias to be kindest to those we know best
through social courtesies to ensure
harmonious relationships with those they
know and interact with daily.*

CHRISTINA GROSS-LOH
PARENTING WITHOUT BORDERS: SURPRISING LESSONS
PARENTS AROUND THE WORLD CAN TEACH US

With anxious concern for her preterm son, a Japanese-American pharmacist listens attentively to pumping instructions. She is alone during our first consult. For the second consult, her husband is at the bedside. There are many questions; they just want to do what's best for their baby, who arrived 6 weeks early.

His will be a brief stay in the NICU, and I tell her one day that she can begin to offer the breast during her visits. We always recommend this before beginning to offer a bottle. It's another three days before I see her again at her baby's bedside, and checking the chart, realize that the baby is only receiving formula.

"What's going on?" I ask, but she only says she left her milk at home. When I also read that she'd not started breastfeeding, I offer to help. Reserved in mannerisms, she declines. I ask how much milk she's making at each pump session, and she reports that it's over 2 ounces, eight times per day. This is a decent supply, well over the baby's current need at any given feeding. I sit down and ooh-and-ah over her son as she holds him nested in her arms, smiling serenely. Another week passes before I see her again. I pick up the chart to read and learn he is still only receiving formula, and she's never offered the breast.

Some mothers feel awkward holding their small babies, and others are anxious about breastfeeding because they can't "see" what's going in. I sit down to understand her situation and see if together we might problem-solve. "Are you changing your mind about breastfeeding? It's okay if you're feeling overwhelmed." There is a shimmer beginning to well in the corner of her eyes.

"My mother is here from Japan for the next 12 months. She says it's not healthy to give my milk until the yellow color is gone." By this, she means colostrum, which is plentiful in the early days, but actually present, and can tinge the milk yellow for up to 2 weeks. I remember reading that there are 42 cultures that consider colostrum taboo. I've just never come across one; nor did I expect it to include the modernized country of Japan. I wrongly assumed this folklore was told in developing countries only. Folktales can pass down from many generations, as it must have in this situation, and I surmise that there are likely many things each of us carry, knowingly and not, from past generations; some things that serve us and some that constrain us.

I sympathize and try to explain the benefits of this *liquid gold*, but she only shakes her head. "I can't go against my mother; she's living with us. I'll work on breastfeeding once the baby is home." Tears pour down her cheeks now, like the 14 days of milk she's been pouring down the drain.

There is no fixing her dilemma. Her mother never visits the hospital and does not speak English. The baby is discharged without having human milk or having breastfed, and she was never able to establish breastfeeding at home. Cultural sensitivity required me to defer to the mother's decision, even as she deferred to her own mother's dictum. In her mind, she realized her mother's understanding of colostrum was untrue, but there were stronger forces at play here than the mind.

The Mother of Premature Twins with a Mind of Her Own

In all affairs, it's a healthy thing now and then, to hang a question mark on the things you have long taken for granted.

BERTRAND RUSSELL

Some mothers don't take our recommendations seriously. And perhaps, it's understandable. When there isn't a definitive answer, and we aren't sure what to recommend, in the medical field, we use the phrase, "the best available evidence leads us to recommend ..." I wonder if this is the case when we make recommendations to mothers about how much straight breast milk their preterm infant should receive each day after discharge (either by bottle or from the breast), and how frequently their milk should have added fortifiers to enhance protein, calcium, and phosphorus, given by bottle. At one point, the experts said they should have the added fortifiers until a baby weighs 3,500 grams (about 7 pounds, 12 ounces). Now, they say this should continue for 9 months. Unfortunately, this new recommendation all but eliminates the possibility of exclusive, direct breastfeeding. I can't bear to say that to a mom who has exclusivity as her goal. I should add that I am oversimplifying this guide. There are many considerations that go into the final discharge recommendation—birthweight, discharge weight, mom's supply, the calories needed to achieve adequate growth, to name a few. But I deflect the question by telling moms that their own pediatrician will direct the decision of when to stop fortifiers after discharge.

Often, the mothers are only able to be in the unit to breastfeed, once or twice per day. So we discharge them not really having seen how they might perform at the breast when they are nursing four to six times per day. As a result, we usually ask that they ease into more frequent nursing, suggesting that for an otherwise healthy preterm baby being discharged over 2,000 grams (4 pounds, 4 ounces), they begin by nursing every other feeding. Even then, they are offered a bottle afterward to assure that they've gotten enough. When they see their pediatrician, which is usually within 2 days, the doctor increases the frequency to 4 to 6 times each day, or so we hope. Eventually, these babies are breastfeeding all but once or twice per day, when they receive fortified milk. We've tracked premature babies closely after discharge and know that most of them only gradually begin to transfer more milk with each breastfeeding session. Once they near their original due date, or at times, a few weeks later, they are often drinking enough from the breast that offering a supplement afterward is unnecessary.

One particular mother of very low birthweight twins (born less than 3 pounds, 5 ounces) made it a point to visit for 3-to-4 hour stretches–long enough to breastfeed each baby once per day. This was impressive, given the juggling she was doing with her schedule to accommodate her other school-aged children. This mom was easy-going and felt perhaps more confident than warranted about how well her premature babies were nursing. They were eager at the breast, but afterward took a full ounce, nearly the volume when solely bottle-fed. It seemed as though she considered them only a few days early instead of 10 weeks early. At discharge, she was given the same guide mentioned above–every other feeding, offer the breast, then the supplement afterward. Essentially, this would mean that one of them was breastfeeding every time, or she could begin nursing simultaneously to save time. She'd had some luck with this prior to discharge, but one baby was less proficient with the initial latch and she usually preferred to nurse one at a time. They went home together on a Thursday. I called to check in about a week after their discharge.

"They're great," she said, with utter confidence, at my inquiry.

"And how did the doctor's appointment go?" I queried.

"Well, they didn't see him last Friday."

"Really? What happened?"

"Well, he has two offices and I thought your discharge coordinator had made the appointment at the Erlanger office and when I got there at 4 in the afternoon, it wasn't even open on Friday. By the time I figured out it must have been scheduled at the other office, it was too late in the day to go."

"So then did you call Monday and get in?"

"No, I haven't gotten around to calling yet. I've been so busy."

I am somewhat alarmed with this news, but felt confident that the babies were fine because even when the babies breastfed, she's supposed to offer a bottle afterward.

"And how's the breastfeeding going?"

"Great," she says, with enthusiastic confidence. "They seem to eat around the clock."

"How so?"

"Well, someone's always on my boob."

"You're nursing 4 times per day, every other feeding, right?

"Nope, they're just breastfeeding."

My heart quickens. "But you give them a bottle afterward to make sure their tummies are full, right?"

"Nope, just the breast, they're doing great—really great."

So much for the best-laid plans. I begin to ask questions and learn that they aren't pooping much, and are at times hard to keep awake to eat, yet she's sure things are going fine. I'm not reassured. Seeing the discharge coordinator walking out of a nearby pod, I wave her over. I'd written down the gist of the conversation and her eyes go buggy. "Ask her if she can take the babies in today."

"Yes, but I don't have an appointment."

Within minutes, an appointment was made through the coordinator, and we were saying our good-byes as she needed to prep the kids to get out the door, into their two car seats, and make it to the pediatricians within the hour.

We heard their growth had indeed faltered, but not drastically, and it was not consequential long-term. How long would she have kept to her routine had I not called is anyone's guess. Same goes for how long it would have taken her to get around to making that pediatrician appointment. I can only say I was thankful I'd called and she'd picked up. The mom, on the other hand, likely thought nothing of it.

I think of breast milk as an amazing best food for all babies, but my experience, and the *best available evidence*, tells me that exclusive breastfeeding is a more distant goal for these twins, whose mother thought otherwise.

Fighting for Their Lives

Medical Transports

And if you have children,
when they cry, does it not stir
something deep inside you?

VICTOR HUGO

THE HUNCHBACK OF NOTRE-DAME

The parents had flown in from Georgia straight from the OB office. No extra clothes, nothing but their two iPads. She was 25 weeks along in her pregnancy of twins when the diagnosis of twin-to-twin transfusion made this trip emergent. But by the time they arrived in Labor and Delivery, the recipient twin fetus had already expired, though her sister would survive and return with her parents to their hometown near Atlanta, 120 days later. The sole stipulation for the discharge was that they would not make this 7-hour trip back home in one day. They stopped several times, any time their daughter cried. A few weeks after arriving home, we shipped all the frozen milk that couldn't be sent home in their car. It was as though, over the 4-month stay, her body was still trying to feed twins. The mom emailed me a picture with a thank you note. The upright deep freezer they purchased was filled to the max with her milk.

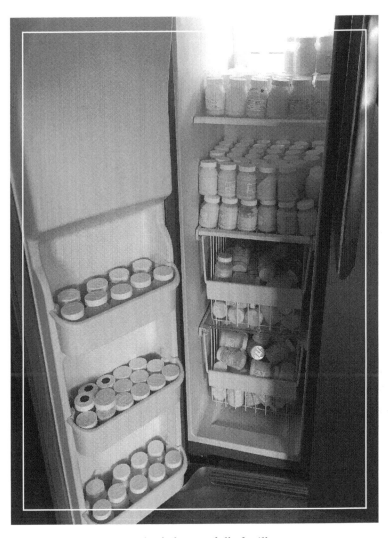

Heather's freezer full of milk

The Dying Baby Who Rallied

The moment we cease to hold each other, the moment we break faith with one another, the sea engulfs us, and the light goes out.

JAMES BALDWIN
NOTHING PERSONAL

How do you support a mother whose tiny, extremely low birthweight baby won't survive? She'd been pumping because we'd asked her. This is why about 20% of the women are pumping for their babies in our NICU. Someone asked. Her baby, TT, whom she nicknamed with affection, was born over 15 weeks early, weighing under a pound. A week or so after his birth, I saw screens around his incubator, and moved forward toward the area. The baby's nurse stopped and cautioned me that he was passing away, and mom was holding him for the first and last time. I proceeded to go behind the screens to offer a few awkward words of comfort. There would be enough time later to talk about her milk supply. As the morning wore on, the screens remained.

By midafternoon, after 4-and-a-half hours of holding her baby, the mom told the nurse she had to leave for an hour to get her 11-year-old daughter from school. I think everyone believed the baby would have already expired that morning, but certainly when she left. With delicate moves, the nurse and respiratory therapist helped transfer TT from his mother's chest back into the incubator. But in a turn of event, almost immediately after she left, TT began to rally. His oxygen levels had never reached this high. If he could maintain them, it was a range clearly compatible with life.

Mom returned to a whole different scenario. The alarms weren't going off constantly. TT was wiggling a bit. She laid her hand on his back, and for the first time had hope.

TT is 4-years-old now. The staff has seen him and his mom often as of late because his now 15-year-old sister has a low birthweight baby in the unit.

The Hawaiian Connection

Fighting Against All Odds

---

*We cannot tell what may happen to us in the
strange medley of life. But we can decide what
happens in us, how we take it, what we do with
it—and that is what really counts in the end.*

JOSEPH FORT NEWTON

She is struggling to hold her baby, to slide him down her shirt. It's only her second time visiting him. I walk over, introduce myself, and help her position the baby for some skin-to-skin contact, and as she begins to speak, her story unfolded like a full-page newspaper. Gaia has a 3- and 4-year-old that flew with her and her husband from Hawaii in March. I sit down. This seems like it's going to be a complicated story, yet she is unusually effervescent as she speaks.

When her second son, Jac, started having intermittent fevers, and periods of lethargy that were unexplainable, she took him in for an evaluation. The physical exam and even the blood tests came back negative; she kept pushing for further testing. Her gut told her something wasn't right. They went between general practitioner and specialist several times; still nothing, and yet, she pressed. At one point, they told her to wean the child because he was allergic to her milk. That made no sense to her, since he'd been growing on it for so many months prior to other symptoms. After several months, more testing was done, and her son's diagnosis was finally made. Jac was suffering from the rarest of childhood cancers. Striking males only, XLP (X-chromosome linked Lymphoproliferative disease) is a disease that affects one in one million children. The average age of onset is 2.5 years, and nearly 75% of the children do not reach their 10th birthday. It's often referred to as an inflammatory storm. She looks for my response as she explains that she breastfed him long-term solely to build his immune system, the very system where he is deficient. "Great intuition and what commitment," I remark. "This was the best thing you could have done for the long road ahead, wasn't it?" She offers a "Thanks be to God," and asks me to help her move her chair into a further reclined position while she holds her preemie close.

They were referred to a hospital in Cincinnati for a bone marrow transplant. This is a complete upheaval in anyone's life, and it happens too often to people traveling across the states and the globe for the best care for their child. There's the worry about the outcome, the cost, leaving home, no income, and no family support, to name a few.

With obvious trepidation, they arrive here in the Queen City in March, 2015. The transplant is postponed several times, which prompts them to finally decide to purchase a car to give them some freedom of movement while here. Then, the week before Jac's 3rd birthday, in December, the procedure was successfully completed. She weaned him shortly before this, partly because she was due to deliver their 4th child in mid-March.

It was important that Jac not be exposed to germs, and the doctors' recommended postponing travel for one month.

Her son would be wearing a protective mask when out in public for a few more months. They sold the car and prepared to fly home mid-January—until her water broke. She delivered their 3rd son eight weeks early. Their journey has been every bit as complicated, and more Odysseus, than I'd ever suspect from the way she speaks with such calm.

A few days later, we are Skyping while I'm visiting with daddy, who's holding the baby in the NICU and big brothers get to see their new sibling. The boys and mommy are only a couple blocks away at the Ronald McDonald House. Her sons sit still only a minute to say hello. In that brief encounter, I only saw rambunctious siblings, not one healthy and one unhealthy son. Mom had a few questions about building her supply, we said our good-byes, and she continued her Skype session with dad.

Think about it. What would it be like being confined to the small space of one room in temporary housing, far from everything familiar—except the husband and sons whom you hold dear? While they look forward to returning to Hawaii, they'd given up an apartment there to travel here, so they will be staying in a room with his mother, she explains pensively. There would be more room at her mother's, but she is on a different island than the children's hospital. Proximity to the hospital will dictate the housing.

I can't adequately explain the sense of privilege it is to walk a short leg of the journey with this family. Their journey has been walked in faith and fueled by prayer.

Unfounded Assumptions

*When something is important enough, you do it
even if the odds are not in your favor.*

ELON MUSK

On a Saturday morning, I am asked to see a mom on the Mother-
Baby unit. Her preterm baby was in the NICU. Mom was just
transferred from the SICU, two days after the birth. Reading her
chart before going in, I note that her BMI is in excess of 50 and
she has a history of low thyroid. Now, just fresh from a critical
event after the birth, she's pumping in room 3361. I've seen so few
moms with a high BMI have a good milk supply that I have little
hope for this working out.

As I enter, she's using the pump. Her eyes brighten, and she
greets me, "Hi, Miss Chris! I was askin' about you yesterday,
but they said you were off." There is a 4-year-old lying on his
belly on the couch coloring away. "You remember Keshaun?"
And while I don't, I go over and squat next to him and greet
him. You can't tell, but he had to be premature. There's no way
she'd remember me otherwise. "He was a 24-weeker. Say hey
to Miss Chris, Keshaun." He raises his head briefly and grins.

"Cool Batman picture," I muse, as his smile widens, showing
sparkling teeth in a perfect row. I wrongly assumed I'd worked
to help her build her supply to no avail. "How long did you end
up pumping?" I ask. Mentally, I'm thinking 2 to 3 weeks, max.
It's discouraging to only get drops time after time. But to my

surprise, she says, "Well, I pumped for the 4 months he was in the hospital, but I had enough milk saved up for another 2 months." I am blown away and my unfounded bias is revealed. She now pulls the bottle out from under her gown. She's single pumping because her breasts are too big to manage pumping simultaneously. This is before we have *hands-free* bras available for moms. But honestly, I don't think the largest of the four sizes would fit her. The bottle is nearly full, just under two ounces.

"Is this the second side? I ask."

"No, ma'am, about to do that next." We return to the conversation about her 4-year-old, as she fastens a lid to the bottle and I attach a new bottle to the shield.

"Any luck getting Keshaun to the breast?"

"You and me tried a lot, but it never went that well. I kept tryin' at home though. We did what we could."

Indeed, they did. This was a good reminder not to make assumptions about potential success based on bias instead of data. While research tells us that moms with a higher BMI may be less likely to breastfeed, it hasn't told us that those who do will have a problem with supply.

Chapter Thirteen

ADULTS IN INTENSIVE CARE

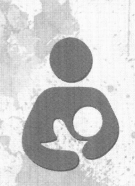

H1N1 - Swine Flu

*Think occasionally of the suffering of which
you spare yourself the sight.*

ALBERT SCHWEITZER

In 2009, I am called to the adult ICU to see a mother who'd delivered, and is unconscious and on a ventilator. Speaking to the staff, I learn that she had nearly succumbed to the H1N1 virus. Her preterm infant is in our NICU. H1N1 was pandemic in the spring of 2009, and pregnant women are at higher risk for developing complications. In a two-month period, there were 45 deaths reported to the CDC; six of them were pregnant women. H1N1 poses additional risk of complications including pneumonia, shortness of breath, respiratory distress, respiratory failure, and death. It's transmitted by air-borne particles in direct contact with hands.

The mother in the ICU remained unconscious for six days. How did they know if she'd want to pump milk for her infant? After all, the emergency birth by cesarean-section was decided on in hopes of at least saving the baby. On morning rounds, three days later, among the dozen or so health care professionals discussing her case is a pharmacist who raises the question, "She's Hispanic, won't she want to pump?" They speak to her husband and learn she'd breastfed three children. There is some skepticism and strong reservations among her care providers. She is literally knocking on death's door. To date, no pregnant woman in acute respiratory failure with H1N1 has survived in the U.S. The decision to proceed lay with the mother's attending physician who consults with our perinatologist and the director of the infection control department.

Not a risk-taker by nature, I arrive in the adult ICU, and carefully consider whether to enter her room. I decide it's safest for my other patients if I assist her at the *end* of the day, when I won't be returning to the maternity ward. I would be less than transparent if I say I don't feel afraid to enter the isolation room, despite being gowned, masked, and gloved like an astronaut. It's a daunting task, and it will be another two days before mom is even conscious. She is the *first* pregnant victim in the U.S. to survive this pandemic.

Like clockwork, her breasts give milk from my first attempt to express them. She remains in the ICU throughout her 14-day stay. Her preterm son is off oxygen before she is even conscious.

Manuel stays longer than her, growing and becoming proficient at eating while his mom lay in isolation, one floor down. She sees him only once during her hospitalization, and this is just as she is being discharged. After this, she stays home many days, still recuperating and pumping on her own.

When she visits Manuel in the NICU, Pod D, bed one, she always brings in milk, but it's rarely much. She never feels up to pumping the recommended 8 times per day, for obvious reasons. Over the next two weeks, until his discharge, she nurses her son during most visits, and then supplements afterward with formula.

I don't know if she was ever able to build a full supply once the baby went home, though it seems unlikely. Still, I've been surprised by some mothers' determination and the body's ability to rebound. Anyone seeing her there, nursing in the pod, would have assumed she was like any mother with a healthy, uneventful delivery of a preemie. Among the baby's caretakers, I was the sole witness to her deteriorated state in the ICU. This gave me a different perspective and admiration of Manuel's mama.

If I had said that the pediatrician's in the NICU didn't think it was in the *mother's* best interest to pump for her preemie, given her critical status, the adult ICU staff would have very likely accepted it without a second thought. I was glad I paused to consider the situation, swallowed my anxiety, and showed up for the lactation consult *her doctor* decided to order.

The Jet Ski Accident

The value of life is revealed when it confronts death from close quarters.

APOORVE DUBEY

Generally, through the years we have only provided lactation coverage 6 days a week. I used to tell the physician interns that they were the breastfeeding consultants in our absence on Sundays, in hopes both the men and women would roll their sleeves up and become proactively involved. When a holiday landed on a Monday, I began a tradition in the mid-90s of covering on Sunday so that there would never be two consecutive days without lactation consultants available.

On this particular Sunday in 2009, I am paged by the operator. Answering, she transfers the call to the Neuro ICU, where a nurse is eager to talk. Her unconscious patient is a young woman in her late 20s who was in a Jet Ski accident the day prior. It's her husband who asks about pumping for their 7-month-old, though surely the staff noticed that she'd been leaking already. When I arrive, supplies in hand, I'm greeted by her nurse who leads me into the room. No family is present. No photos, no flowers, only the mother who lies in the bed attached to monitors, while the nurse speaks to me in the hushed tones I consider reserved for poor outcomes.

I teach the nurse how to use the pump, how to label and store the milk, who to call for questions about the compatibility of any new medications she might be prescribed, how long the milk is safe, and the availability of the lactation department staff. The nurse herself had breastfed two children many years earlier, but she'd never needed to pump. She is off to tend to her another patient while I stay at the bedside another 20 minutes to complete the pumping. I talk to the unresponsive mom as I work.

"I hear you have two kiddos." *Pause.* She shows no sign she hears me, but I persist. "I'm gonna ask your nurse to have your husband bring pictures in. I'd love to see them. They'll be a good visual motivator during your rehab, too." *Pause.* "You have a lot to fight for to get back to your old self, Natalie. But 'til then, let your breasts and your milk will be your link to home and family, huh?" *Pause.*

After transferring four partially filled bottles of expressed milk into three full bottles, I sit down, hold her hand just barely at her fingertips, and wait for her nurse. Our breathing is all I focus on as I sit in silence and wait. The return of the function of this mother's extremities is not guaranteed. I never asked about the prognosis because I didn't want to hear. It's likely a self-protective stance, I know. But it's a coping strategy too—for now, I'd just rather stick to a hoping strategy.

As with many of my patients, I am there at a moment in their lives and not beyond, rarely knowing what comes of them. But in this moment, we are together.

The Mother in
the Tilt-a-Whirl Bed

*You don't utilize that bed unless a person is
knocking on death's door.*

ANNIE

CRITICAL CARE NURSE

She is prone, belly down, unconscious, facing the floor, facing off death just after the birth of her daughter. When I am called to the adult ICU, I rarely know ahead of time what I may come upon. Stroke victim? Boating accident victim? Burn victim? Regardless, they're always critical. Today, it is an upside-down mother. It's obvious, logistically-speaking that I won't be setting her up to pump for now.

When I ask to speak to her nurse, I'm approached by a bustling RN, who immediately asks why I am there. My badge does not signal my occupation, as it says only "nurse clinician." I preface by saying I work in the newborn ICU and have just come from the baby's bedside. I'm hoping this will ease what I say next. "I'm the breastfeeding consultant."

I understand ICU nurses. They are territorial and fiercely protective of their patients, a quality I admire. I underestimate how she will react. Nearly jumping back a huge step, she looks at me quizzically as if to say, "You've got to be kidding me!" As she shifts her eyes toward the patient strapped to the tilt-a-whirl bed, I give the nurse a short minute to process the fact that I indeed want to assist with breast pumping—at least, eventually, when the roto-prone bed shifts the mother upright and she's deemed stable enough. But for now, she's in acute respiratory distress, from pulmonary hypertension. The mother is carefully strapped in, while the bed rotates a complete 360-degree circle, shifting fluids away from her lungs where they've been building up. Despite the high maternal mortality rate after births in the U.S., I've seen so few mothers' die after birth, I'm probably overly optimistic that this mother will survive. Clearly, the nurse doesn't share my optimism because she's been caring for the mother since the delivery.

I tell the nurse that the doctors have asked me to assess the feasibility of expressing the mother's milk. She explains that the mother is critical, that over half of women who deliver with a diagnosis of pulmonary hypertension don't make it. I assure her that I understand and let her know I'll report back to the physician caring for the mother's extremely low birthweight infant.

Two more days go by and Chris, our attending neonatologist, aware the mother is still alive, asks me to go with her to pay the patient and ICU staff a visit. When a mother is critically ill, her milk doesn't always come in, or often comes in late or in small quantities. At times, this is secondary to medicines she's received while in a critical state. I've also seen milk come in as late as 11 days after a birth instead of the usual 72 hours. I've no idea what this mom's lactation potential is.

Coming into the unit, Chris sees her counterpart in the adult world. The ICU attending doc has just finished rounds and is giving her residents the day's parting instructions. Chris approaches the group and introduces herself with the confidence of a seasoned physician. The team perks up, interested to learn the status of the premature infant. Then she comes around to the question of pumping the mother, but before anyone can object, she builds a case for how removing milk, could actually help the mother's condition, alleviating the strain of added fluid (milk) and the swelling associated with severe engorgement from around the mother's lungs. The physician is cautiously entertaining this as an added therapeutic approach to the mother's care. In the end, the mother's doctor agrees, but asks our neonatologist to sign a legal document stating that expressing milk is in the mother's (and obviously the baby's) best interest. Once she does this, I introduce myself to the new nurse caring for the mother. She's upright now, but I have no supplies with me. This nurse has breastfed her own children and is receptive to the education and reassurances she is receiving from Chris. We agree that I'll return within the hour to initiate pumping while the mom is still in an upright position.

Milk pours out like a crack in a child's plastic swimming pool, steadily draining. We have collected over three ounces, as the mother lies motionless on the bed. I speak to her as though she were wide awake, telling her how cute her baby is, and letting her know we look forward to her first visit to the NICU. It's days before I meet a quasi-alert mother, who, though not yet speaking, seems happy that I'm pumping her, half-smiling as she watches the milk empty into the bottles, once I've moved her oily, long brown hair off her chest so she can see.

The father of the baby tells us she'd wanted to breastfeed all along. She can't speak for herself yet, so his rather talkative and assertive demeanor doesn't surprise me. Over time, the ICU staff tells me he hardly lets her speak, even when she can. Still, I don't know if this results from a sense of overprotection. Over the coming days, I can see that her family is reserved in his presence. He looks about 15 years her senior, which may play a factor.

Remarkably, as mom becomes more stable, she continues to make ever-increasing volumes of milk. Dad is vigilant in insisting the ICU staff help with pumping every three hours around the clock, until the two of them can manage it on their own. His forcefulness doesn't endear him, but I have to admit that she probably pumps twice as often with his advocating. When she is considered fully out of the woods, she makes a wheelchair visit to the NICU, several bottles of milk in hand. We switch her from the two-ounce bottles to larger four-ounce bottles, to make pumping easier and to get a nice mix of calories in all bottles. Dad has been holding their daughter in mother's absence, but she now sheds her gown and blissfully holds her daughter skin to skin.

Dad continues speaking for mom throughout the baby's hospitalization, only relenting when the nurses say, "We'd like mom to answer this question, if that's OK with you." Over time, they learn the art of breastfeeding together and the baby is discharged home partially breastfeeding and partially receiving her mother's expressed milk that is fortified with added protein, minerals, and calories.

Eight months after discharge, two lactation consultants drive 45 minutes to a neighboring county to participate in a fair sponsored by the county's WIC department. This family strolls up to the booth, mother holding her baby in a sling and breastfeeding as she walks. Dad begins his own PR blurb, attributing the survival of the mother and baby to the staff of UCMC. It's rewarding to overhear these stories, and today we're glad he's such an extrovert!

Several months after this, we receive an email from the WIC nutritionist assigned to their county. She tells us that dad is singing the praises of the lactation staff who came to their rescue when she couldn't speak for herself, and when he didn't know there was a way to preserve breastfeeding. She reiterates that they are grateful for the LCs who started mom on the path of nursing. The parents had been in for a well-baby check, she was still breastfeeding, still quiet in the dad's presence, but healthy–and alive. Alive!

Chapter Fourteen

MEMORIES OF LOSS

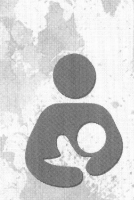

SIDS

I didn't want to kiss you goodbye that was the trouble; I wanted to kiss you goodnight. And there's a lot of difference.

ERNEST HEMINGWAY

In my first month as a lactation consultant, I went into room 3350 to see a mother who'd just returned from her tubal ligation. Kelly was in her early 20s, and this was her second child. I casually commented about her unusual permanent decision at such a young age. She replied with confidence, describing sterilization as a decision she made with certitude. She'd bottle-fed her other child, but knowing this was her last, she wanted to breastfeed. It's a mindset I often encounter. The baby, born 3 and a half weeks early, was a natural, proficient mammal. She held him in a football hold that afternoon, an easy way to keep her large breasts away from his nose, as well as keep his weight off her new, small incision.

Kelly mentioned that she was going to be discharged after supper on the same day as the surgery, instead of the next morning. This was something else I found highly unusual, but it was at her request. She was anxious to get to grandma's house, show off the baby, and pick up her older daughter. I know tubals are considered minor surgery, but I cautioned her not to overdo it. The consult lasted a mere 20 to 25 minutes. The baby nursed like a champ.

Eleven days later, I was paged by the director of neonatology. Yes, I remembered the mom. Yes, I'd observed breastfeeding. What's this about, I wondered, as the story unfolded. They'd stayed late at grandma's, gotten the kids bedded down, and Kelly wasn't in bed herself until after midnight. About 4 a.m., the baby, who was sleeping in a bassinet at her side, awoke for a feeding. She breastfed, fell asleep, not sure how long, but awoke and lay the baby back in the bassinet. Within the hour, she startled awake, reached for her baby, to find he wasn't breathing. Her husband called 911, while she attempted to give rescue breaths. The baby was pronounced dead on arrival.

It was difficult for the neonatologist and OB medical director to meet with the parents. In the course of the meeting, they offered to reverse the mother's tubal ligation. The final autopsy report would be forthcoming, but at this initial consult, they didn't discuss with Kelly and her husband what the preliminary findings showed.

There was a confluence of risk factors for SIDS in this case: exhausted mother on pain medicine, falling asleep with baby in arms, larger breasts, and a slightly preterm infant. An experience like this, especially this early in my lactation career, shaped how I speak to parents, what I say, emphasize, and reiterate about safe sleep. It also led me to the extensive research of Dr. James McKenna, Director of the Mother-Baby Behavioral Sleep Laboratory at The University of Notre Dame. He has published specific recommendations for safe sleep. One tragedy is one tragedy too many.

Lessons from a Social Worker

When we die, we go into the arms of those
who remember us.

ROSIE MALEZER

In 2006, I attended a Nursing Grand Rounds lecture, but learned more in the 15 minutes after the presentation than during the presentation itself. Topics for these lectures are vastly different: care of surgical incisions, cultural sensitivity, and advanced nursing practices, to name a few. I've only attended this monthly series twice: both of the topics were obstetric-related. The presentation isn't memorable, or perhaps it is simply overshadowed by what transpires after. When it was over, a middle-aged woman in street clothes and a lab coat, a social worker I would learn, approached me and greeted me by name.

"You helped me breastfeed my son 8 years ago." Oh, dear, I think, another mother whom I can't remember. On the other hand, a woman's memory surrounding birth can be amazing. After this introduction, another story unfolds; I suspect the one she really wants me to know.

Eight years prior, I'd helped her initiate pumping during her two-day stay after delivering a critical baby who was immediately transferred to the NICU. He passed away in her arms the day after her own discharge. With no baby to receive her milk, it didn't occur to her to use her pump to relieve her ever-tightening breasts. She knew our office hours ended at 5 in the evening, and by late evening, she tells me she was now aching physically as well as emotionally. After several calls, her husband finally reached a La Leche League leader at 1 in the morning. He was told to purchase a head of green cabbage, press out the leaves to get the juices flowing, and then wrap them around his wife's breasts. Though just as distraught as his wife, he went out to find a 24-hour grocery and purchase the cabbage. As I listen, I am saddened that they weren't advised to use the ice that was right in their freezer, known to be equally effective as the juice of cabbage.

The poor husband misunderstood the instructions, or perhaps, if they were expressed as I've described, the instructions were so vague that "press" could easily have been misconstrued. The League leader could have said to use the side of a coffee cup and roll it over the leaves until the juices of the cabbage were flowing. Instead he took her literally and went directly to the basement laundry room, set up the iron, and *pressed* the leaves. Though he scorched some, her husband took the remaining leaves up to the bedroom and she applied them around her breasts. She had no relief from her engorgement or her grief, the breast-swelling worsening by the hour. In the early morning hours, she phoned a friend who was breastfeeding and who suggested she wrap ice in towels and place the towels on her breasts. Later the friend arrived with a shoulder to cry on and food for dinner.

There were no tears as the social worker relayed her story to me, only the request that I develop a hand-out for mothers who may be in a similar situation in the future. I did so immediately. Today, that hand-out is part of the NICU bereavement packet.

On the Circuit with
the *Curves* Coach

*Regret is a sad, harsh feeling when we fail to
do something our heart wanted to do.*

ANURAG PRAKASH RAY

It's early evening and I'm on the circuit at *Curves* within an hour of closing. As the music booms in the background the coach is talking about her full-time job. She's a music teacher. She's shared enough for me to know she has a lot on her plate with two jobs and a husband who's developed early-onset Alzheimer's. She turns and asks what I do for a living.

"I'm a lactation consultant up at UC hospital," I say during the upswing on a piece of equipment.

Immediately, she is holding her hand to her chest, saying, "Ah, my heart, I tried so hard and failed." She clutches her chest this way through the entire conversation and moans aloud at intervals.

I surmise that her child has to be over 10 by now, yet still she carries the disappointment with her like it was yesterday. Feeling for her, and to lift the air, I ask if he survived infancy.

"Well, yeah," she says, chuckling aloud.

"Give yourself a break, Diane. I'm sure you did the best you could under the circumstances." I don't even have to ask what those circumstances were because she's pouring her heart out as I finish my sentence.

"I didn't have milk, I had bleeding nipples, and they were flat to start with...and I got mastitis with a temperature of 105! And I had a red streak right up here," as she point to her left collar bone. It's a litany of worst-case scenarios.

"Good grief, that's terrible," I say in all sincerity.

"I cried and cried, I was so sad," and she trails off. After a reflective pause, she adds, "They sent me home in 24 hours–I had no idea what I was doing, and the home nurse came out and said I had the worst nipples ever."

"Oh my gosh! It sounds like such a stressful start to being a mom. I'm so sorry."

"And she had me pump and you know back then those pumps weren't worth a dime. I gave him milk for two weeks, well, that and some formula."

"You really, really struggled. A lot of moms don't know that the colostrum is mixed in with mature milk for a whole two weeks, so you gave him lots of antibodies."

"Really?" she asks with a pause, hand still over heart. "I was so sad, so disappointed."

"You struggled so much." I wait before asking, "How old is he now?"

"Twenty-two."

"You were a good mom."

"Thanks."

Memories surrounding birth and feeding can last a life time, for better and worse. I hope we've improved our support to moms and are better at helping them through closure when needed. There was no hint of guilt in her story. This is regret at how something unfolded–at something *her heart wanted to do*. I understand that. I hope all of us understand that.

Chapter Fifteen

CLOSE TO HOME
THE NEIGHBORHOOD

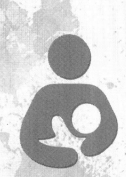

The Courthouse Encounter

My work as a lactation consultant intertwines with my life outside the hospital, creating a tapestry of relationships that begin in unexpected places.

We sit in the hallway of the courthouse on an uncomfortable wooden bench, me and my 6-year-old son. Next to us is a couple with their 6-year-old. It's awkward to meet them under these circumstances, but Jackie and Jeff Senior introduce themselves and chat away with ease, their voices echoing off the high ceilings of the hall.

Andrew and Jeff Junior met a few weeks earlier while biking at a nearby playground. Two boys demanded they hop off their bikes. Both bikes were Christmas presents, and they were enjoying their very first ride, as signs of spring were breaking. The boys gave up their bikes to the strangers who made off with them. Andrew's Aunt Mary would tell us later, a brokenhearted

Andrew told her, "My bike is my life." Meanwhile, Jeff Sr. called the police. The offenders were found, and the police pressed charges.

Jackie rants on about justice while our boys sit in silent worry. There is something charming about this thin, 5'10" street-wise woman with long straight, brown hair who inserts my name into every other sentence like an essential punctuation mark. Yet, as tough as she talks in the hallway, Jackie's demeanor changes when we're called into the judge's chamber to sit down with the offenders and their mothers. She listens to their story of trying to raise children in the projects. She speaks with compassion, talking to the mothers about her own experience being a single, teen mom. With calm reassurance, she tells them she understands how tough that job is.

"It's damn hard work, I should know. And my parents were no help whatsoever." Even the judge leans forward, intent to listen.

"I tell Jeff all the time, I don't know how I made it through before he came into my life." But my girls were in grade school by then. Jeff smiles, says nothing, and nods in agreement. He doesn't seem taken by surprise when his wife, who seemed hellbent on retribution just 15 minutes prior, speaks with such kindheartedness now. The two mothers, nodding as well, listen in silence. I think this must be the meaning of mercy. We don't know what the outcomes for the boys were once we left the chambers. Andrew and I parted ways with Jeffrey and his parents. I would have never guessed we'd have a long relationship after this encounter.

I have seen Jackie a few times at the hospital while she's visiting new grandchildren, and we catch up on the boys as I visit with the family. Twenty-five years later, she forwards a lovely tribute on Facebook from her daughter, a compilation of songs playing in the background as photos flip on the screen - her granddaughter, Kylie, from birth through this day, her 10th birthday. Kylie's mom's tribute began, "So 10 *years ago today, I never expected to be a teen mommy...*"

Jackie's post to me reads, "Chris Auer, here is one of your breastfed preemies!!!"

It's both the boys and the grandbabies that have bonded us.

Age and Wisdom

*There's much talk in our society about
motherhood in general, but an awkward silence
surrounds many of the concrete realities.*

TRUDELLE THOMAS
SPIRITUALITY IN THE MOTHER ZONE

I have come to deplore the acronym, AMA, standing for "advanced maternal age." I understand it can create risks in pregnancy, but still, how does that make an older first-time pregnant mom feel? It's defined as someone over 35, not ancient. (Would that I was that young again!) One such "older" neighbor had invited me to her house to talk about breastfeeding. In 1992, the term was "elderly primip," meaning older mother, first-time pregnancy. We visited while she was on bedrest during the final two months of her pregnancy. The timing coincided with the early months of my hospital establishing a lactation department, yet was still before I had a formal lactation credential behind my name.

Trudelle was 39 when she became pregnant, 40 when she delivered. Our birthdays are days apart. She considered every detail around pregnancy, birth, breastfeeding, and child-raising, and had lots of time to read and observe other moms. We reviewed what I review with all expectant mothers regarding what to anticipate after the birth. I used a doll so she could practice positioning, and also examined her breasts. She was as prepared as she could be. Her breastfeeding was initiated with ease and she continued nursing her son for 4 *years*.

When she returned to her position as an English professor, she discovered ways to incorporate insights gained as a mother into a writing course titled, *Writing about Parenting*. Eventually, she wrote the book, *Spirituality in the Mother Zone*, where she explores how motherhood, with all its grit and grime, can lead you on a journey of faith. Her premise, in part, is that by a regular practice of reflecting on your experience as woman and mother, you can awaken to the innate meaning and insights that parenting and your child offer, even in the more harrowing days. I am a believer!

One of her students was the 22-year-old daughter of my long-time friend, Linda. Angela was the first baby I'd ever witnessed breastfeed. She was a senior in Trudelle's class when she gave a presentation titled, *Motherhood in the Trenches*, sharing her experience and pictures from labor and birth through her daughter's 16th month. What a lovely serendipity.

The stories and meaning ascribed to the birth of a mother spread horizontally like rhizomes, as they are told from person to person. Trudelle had the foresight to know this. Wisdom, not just a baby, descends and spreads to others when AMA mothers birth.

Almond Eyes, Protruding Tongue

There are only two lasting bequests
we can hope to give our children; one is
roots and the other is wings.

JOHANN WOLFGANG VON GOETHE

Two-to-four-day hospital stays make for difficult to identify subtle abnormalities in newborns. Though close and early follow-up is needed to assure a baby's well-being, still many clinics and pediatric offices are too busy to see these newborns soon enough. To fill in the gap, home health nurses can be life-savers. By 2000, the number of agencies willing to provide these important visits dwindled due to poorer reimbursement from insurance companies.

In 1990, a singer from our wedding and his wife moved in about eight houses down from ours on Beechwood Avenue. I knew Carol had breastfed Jason, her first, and assumed it had gone smoothly, since I was never approached to discuss any concerns. After the birth of their second child though, a year after I'd become a breastfeeding consultant, she asked if I would come and observe a feeding. Carol wasn't quite sure everything was alright.

Moms can be incredibly astute when noticing even very slight differences between breastfeeding one child compared to another. As we sat and talked before she latched Katie on, one thing was hard to miss. Katie was frequently thrusting her tongue forward, an unusual behavior for a newborn. At the breast, the tongue rolls backward in a wave-like motion to extract milk, so I could see why Carol was struggling. Additionally, a forward tongue thrust can be a sign of Down syndrome. Another common sign is ovoid, or pear-shaped eyes. Katie had both. But did she have the chromosomal abnormality? No. It took Carol a bit of time to find that opportune moment between forward tongue thrusts to latch Katie on, but they found their groove in time.

As I write this, Katie is in her final semester of college, and is using it to study abroad in Vietnam, then post-graduation, she sets off for Alaska as part of the Jesuit Volunteer Corp. The baby girl, who found her own way to nourish, grew up to be the young woman who was using her gifts to explore and contribute to the broader world.

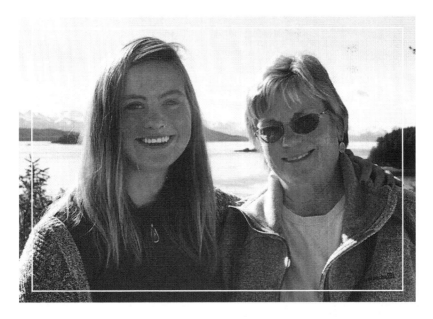

❋ *Katie and Carol in Alaska* ❋

Unintended Presence at
a Home Birth

*A baby is God's opinion that the
world should go on.*

CARL SANDBURG

Jerry and Susan moved in as newlyweds, just two doors down from us. Prior to the wedding, Jerry lived with us for six months after returning from Mexico, where he and his fiancé had been volunteering at homeless shelters. Our daughter, Amy, spent lots of time with them and eventually cared for their firstborn on occasion. So it confused me when Amy came rushing into our bedroom late one night saying Susan had called and needed me to come over because Jerry's cousin was having a baby.

"Why do I have to go over? Why can't you babysit?" I'm in a fog, even as I'm answering her.

"No, mom. I think she's having the baby *at their house.*"

Incredulous, I called Susan. "Yes!! Get over here. They were on the way to the hospital when she felt the urge to push. It was either try to make it the two miles to our house or deliver in the car at the BP station."

"Did you call 911?"

"Yes. Commme."

Christina's Birth

You never know what may be asked of you
by unexpected midnight calls in winter.
you may awake, half-dazed,
fog rolling over REM sleep.

If it's of grave import, you may startle to
attention, don your royal purple night robe,
slide your feet into pink slippers,
race down squeaking stairs into the night.

You might arrive at neighbor's home,
see two men, two women—
one panting, moaning, belly bursting
leaning over kitchen chair.

You may think you are not needed,
a back-up plan, a short-term spectator,
until she's pushing and the silence of the
night tells you no medic will arrive.

You never know what you might say
when adrenaline is pulsing
through your previously tired body
now standing at alert.

When you ask her to lie down,
it must be fear that's talking –
you know full well babies
birth better when mothers squat.

You never know how your heart will race,
rising thuds, beating faster with each contraction
or that your breathing with her
is just as much to calm yourself.

You don't anticipate what you'll think
when head emerges, pale, round—quiet
without the rest of her slender body
sliding through the birth canal.

You hide your panic but wonder
if you are witness to a miracle
or emergency extraordinaire, as you wait—
as two minutes dangle, just like her head.

You want to trust that nature will not choose
this moment to withhold cooperation
or that you will laugh as the man innocently asks:
isn't the rest of the body supposed to come out?

You never know as you kneel and receive her
if you will weep before her first cry,
pass out before the placenta comes,
remember to raise her body higher than the cord.

You wouldn't expect you'd be so mesmerized
watching *this* pink newborn nursing—*this* night
since you put babies to breast
a hundred times a week.

You sit on hardwood floor
bow in reverent awe
intimate witness to this ritual,
ancient—ever new.

A League of Their Own

---

*Yet, isn't it in this inner realm where mothers
really live—facing unfamiliar waves of anxiety,
desire, and uncertainty that accompany each
day with a new baby? ...
New mothers often wonder whether others
are going through a similar upheaval.*

DANIEL STERN & NADIA BRUSCHWEILER-STERN
PEDIATRICIAN AND PSYCHIATRIST
BIRTH OF A MOTHER

There was a period in the mid-90s that our parish, in central Cincinnati, provided meeting space for a La Leche League group. When the church's meeting room was under renovation, I contacted the leader and offered my nearby home as an alternate place to gather. In 1995, the League is very active, and this particular group is a combination of first-time and experienced moms.

I greet the moms as they come for their meeting. The energy is infectious. They are enthused about motherhood in general, and breastfeeding, in particular. Spreading out in my small family room, they sit on the floor, couch, chairs, and loveseat, 10 moms and babes in all. The ages range from 6 weeks to 2 1/2 years. The seven mothers navigate the path of parenthood, freely discussing whatever is on their minds in a safe, judgement-free environment. Two League Leaders facilitate.

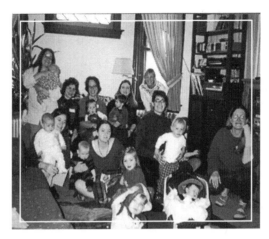

* La Leche League *

On delivery day, more than just babies are born; mothers are born too, a fact all too often underappreciated. I see these moms turn to each other and the leaders for guidance. One mom shares her exasperation with reflux, and takes in advice, then later offers suggestions to another mom who is dealing with uninvited comments from well-intentioned family members. I see them each tentatively assuming this role of mother, learning by osmosis as much as by discussion, forming bonds, seeking out kindred spirits, perhaps making future best friends.

I've read that mothers in developing countries have similar doubts that they are "doing it right," or whether they have enough milk. What they have going for them is a community of experienced women to advise, and the mother's mother. In so many countries, the experienced grandmother hosts the new mom from birth through the first 3-to-6 months of their grandchild's life. This includes India, Nepal, Nigeria, Albania, and Namibia, to name a few. In Denmark, even in the hospital, mothers eat in a communal setting so that they are getting and giving support right from day one. Unlike the U.S., with its minimal post-birth support, in the Netherlands, mothers are given postpartum medical care. A nurse comes daily to help with breastfeeding and assist in household chores, and the midwife provides home visits as well. Many countries, by the way, consider household chores off limits to a new mom for three months.

I am so glad to be home that day, but make a point to stay in the background. I want to learn from them instead of taking my usual role of doling out answers. Playing hostess and serving snacks gives me that opportunity. I have a photo keepsake of the group from that Thursday morning. The League has been a gift for women in search of support and extended family in our transient culture. However, with so many women returning to the workforce, part of their mission is being fulfilled through social media. I treasure the snapshot of their lives that this group of women allowed me to witness.

Special Needs Children
and their Parents

The human spirit is one of ability,
perseverance and courage that no
disability can steal away.

UNKNOWN

In the 1990s, it was quite common for homecare companies to receive reimbursement for a nurse's visit to moms and babes within the first 48 hours of their hospital discharge. I provided staff education for several of these companies and they all had my pager. Late one afternoon, I took a call from a nurse I knew who'd made a home visit in my neighborhood, and was concerned about a 2 1/2-day-old full-term baby who was lethargic when breastfeeding.

I knew the birth history. I'd seen this mother prior to discharge from the hospital during their short 12-hour stay. Mom had breastfed another child for over 2 1/2 years. That alone was encouraging. She was experienced and didn't have a history of low supply. With this second child, she'd gone into labor about 1 in the morning. The mom's urge to push was immediate and couldn't be forestalled. She birthed the baby at home, and went into the hospital immediately afterward.

In the hospital, we make a point to observe babies breastfeeding. However, the timing of this consult had coincided with him just finishing up at the breast. Time didn't allow for further observation prior to their discharge. Because of the mom's history of successful breastfeeding, and the two follow-up home visits by a registered nurse ordered at 24 and 72 hours after discharge, I was not overly concerned that I hadn't observed him feeding.

The most common causes of lethargy include being born prematurely, being underfed, and being moderately jaundiced. Mild jaundice occurs in about 67 percent of all full-term newborns with no consequence. When something occurs in vast numbers like this, clinicians begin to wonder if it has beneficial effects. In fact, in studies, jaundice has been found to aid in brain and eye development, that is, if it remains only mild. This is a huge caveat. High levels, as determined by a blood test, are dangerous. This baby's level was checked and found to be in the mild range. So it was not the reason for his lethargy.

I called the mom after the homecare nurse's call, and she was delighted to have me stop in that very evening. I listened to what she said had been happening as I changed the diaper of her rousing son. Instead of the usual clear to light yellow, the urine in the diaper was tea-color brown. He also hadn't had a poop in over 24 hours—unusual, since breast milk has a laxative effect. There was cause for immediate concern. While he now seemed pretty awake, he latched to the breast in a listless manner and nibbled only briefly. I noted her nipple size and wondered if he'd been sucking on it alone instead of the dark areola surrounding the nipple, where he would more effectively transfer milk. A shallow latch could be a key to understanding his lethargy. If it continued, over time, he'd potentially be drinking inadequate amounts and begin sleeping more for lack of energy to stay awake.

She went hunting for her packed breast pump. What I was seeing was troublesome enough that I decided to proceed with offering the formula the father had given me. Standard practice would have me offer formula with something other than a bottle and artificial nipple in order to avoid exposing her baby to a different texture and tongue movement. Artificial nipples can make some babies reluctant to breastfeed, especially with early, repeated use. At the hospital, we usually use specialized infant cup feeders for short-term supplementation, but I didn't have one at my disposal. I was also concerned that his pattern of disorganized and weak suck could put him at risk for swallowing down the wrong track ("aspiration," in medical jargon). He took the bottle poorly, one to two teaspoons over a 20-minute attempt. His subsequent attempt with his mother's milk yielded no better result. Alarmed, I suggested they take him to the ER. They opted to attempt frequent feedings and see their pediatrician in the morning.

It was a long time and many appointments with specialists before they got to a rare diagnosis, global apraxia, rooted in a neurologic disorder that in part reveals itself in poor motor coordination. When everything else about this baby boy seemed perfect, it took time for his parents to comprehend that their journey with this son would not be the same as his older brother's. Because of advances in technology now, most abnormalities are identified weeks or months in advance of delivery, giving parents much needed time to adjust to a diagnosis and prepare emotionally. It can be devastating to learn that your expectation of a healthy baby isn't accurate. This couple was thrust into a new reality with no preparation. No one wants to enter icy water and have to swim, but swim they did. While still difficult to accept, time to prepare is something

I wish this family had. Today, this well-loved, special needs young man is 21 years old. I see him nearly weekly at church.

The Englishman and Postpartum Depression

*You are okay. You will get better. You will
feel yourself again. You may not believe that's
possible now: Cling to it anyway.*

UNKNOWN

This is the story of the couple I got to know while sharing space in a storage closet. Throughout the 90s, I taught a 90-minute infant care class to new parents, followed by a two-hour breastfeeding class for those who were interested in staying. The classes were well attended by a dozen mothers. A few came alone, some brought their own mothers, but most were accompanied by the father of the baby. I encourage bringing a partner because mothers are notoriously tired after the birth, and tired moms only recall fragments of the class. To help them remember, I developed a 5-by-7 card for the baby's crib using the acronym B.R.E.A.S.T.F.E.D. which highlights nine basic facts about initiating breastfeeding. At times, I wondered if I should just drill down with this card in any number of creative ways and call it a day after 30 minutes of class. Another good reason to have a partner come is that new moms benefit from a cheering gallery through the early days.

At the end of the breastfeeding class, I offered a private one-on-one consult in case the mother wanted to discuss a particular concern she might be inhibited to discuss in the group. It was also a time to offer a breast exam and, based on this, suggest positions to hold the baby that might best work for a mom's given anatomy. It was a time to build confidence. Crazily enough, I held these consults in the only private space available—the walk-in storage closet of the classroom. No one seemed to notice or mind this oddity.

With 20 to 24 people in class, and varying stages of being on board with breastfeeding, I used a lighthearted approach interjected with lots of stories and analogies to illustrate points. There was always some laughter, as well as earnest desire to understand. Inevitably in the Winter, the guys had college basketball on their minds. It was more than one occasion when a dad would suggest that latching a baby quickly when they opened their mouths wide was like slam dunking the basketball. Even the moms roared. Occasionally, I'd have to lasso a dad who'd gone off topic. Participation helps recall, but keeping everyone on topic was an important skill that I honed over time.

At one particular class, I met with a couple after the class. Thomas was a businessman from England when he'd come to the U.S., where he met and married his wife, Celia. They were a darling couple in their mid-20s, and seemed well suited for each other. I don't know their thoughts about returning to England, but I assumed that the baby would be raised in the U.S. Both were educated and enthusiastic about nursing this first-born. I anticipated there may be a learning curve and some discomfort with nursing if no one was with her in the first several attempts. Babies' adrenaline levels are never higher their whole lives than in the very first hour or so after birth. That means even babies whose mothers take painkillers during labor, or whose mother's breasts make breastfeeding difficult—even those babies generally nurse well within the first hour of life.

Unfortunately, Celia was not able to nurse the baby within the first hour because the delivery turned into an emergent cesarean-section that involved general anesthesia. By the time she awoke, the baby had slid into her own deep sleep phase. Subsequent latches were always a struggle with the baby opening her mouth only half as wide as needed, causing a shallow latch. Mom became more tender each day. I spent time with her each of the four days they were hospitalized. Her previous happy countenance was gone. She sank a little lower in mood each day. She was eating sparsely, sliding her fork through her scrambled eggs as though she were sifting for some unreachable treasure.

When we talked about follow-up support, I learned they lived only seven blocks from me. We had not yet established the Lactation Education Resource Center, a clinic where Dr. Ballard and I would come to provide ongoing lactation support. As Celia and baby were discharged, I gave Thomas the number of the pager I wore 24/7. He contacted me about a week later and asked if I could visit. I found a despondent mom who wanted no more to do with breastfeeding. I tried to validate her feelings, and to help dad come to terms with her decision to wean. He still wanted so much for her to breastfeed, despite the fact that he looked exhausted from running the household and providing most of the care for their newborn. A few days later, he called and said Celia was not getting out of bed at all to care for herself or the baby. He was beside himself, not knowing how to motivate her, and not able to take more time off work. It's hard enough when family isn't in town. For them, family was out of state and out of the country. Their earlier joyful anticipation had completely disintegrated. I referred them back to their midwife, who was already scheduled to see Celia the next day for her 2-week checkup.

I didn't have the experience or credentials to distinguish between baby blues and postpartum depression, let alone the more severe postpartum psychosis. Postpartum anxiety wasn't even a term in 1996. And the Edinburgh Postnatal Depression Scale, though published in 1987, was not yet used routinely at the first postpartum doctor/midwife visit. I assumed Celia was going through the mildest version of depression, since many moms are teary in the first week as hormones shift. This happens to about 85% of women after birth, often enough so it's not considered unusual.

Depression affects one in 10 Americans, and according to the Center for Disease Control (CDC) antidepressants are the third most commonly prescribed medications in the U.S. behind cardiovascular drugs and cholesterol-lowering medicines. I recently reviewed the charts of 100 breastfeeding mothers we had seen over a month. I found that 23 percent of the mothers had depression as one of their medical conditions prior to pregnancy, while 17 percent had an anxiety diagnosis, some of which reflect a dual diagnosis. These women are more vulnerable to mood disorders after the birth.

The obstetric staff now screens for depression during the routine postpartum check-up, but this normally doesn't occur until 2 or 6 weeks after birth, sometimes long after a mother has begun to spiral downward. More pediatrician offices are screening mothers sooner since all babies are routinely seen within 2 or 3 days after discharge. When she met with her midwife, Celia was prescribed an antidepressant, but the symptoms likely wouldn't abate for 3 to 4 weeks. I was very happy to hear she was willing to take the medicine, because the persistent taboos about mental health and taking medicine are so pervasive in the U.S. that many mothers try to tough it out month after month, not understanding why they have low energy and feel disconnected from themselves and their babies.

Still, there was damage done to the spousal relationship over those first 8 weeks. It was a heartbreaking situation. Thomas, simply forlorn, called a couple more times over the next two months. I was not hearing anything optimistic. Running into him at the local grocery store several months later, he tearfully told me she was asking for a divorce.

Full Circle

Our First Babysitter

None of us, including me, ever do great things.
But we can all do small things, with great love,
and together we can do something wonderful.

MOTHER TERESA

Sixteen-year-old Kathy was our girls' first babysitter and nearby neighbor, living in the white house with the front porch swing across the street, and just a few houses away.

It's a lovely full-circle moment when you find yourself caring for your babysitter's baby. What I remember about my time with her was something she shared with me when I first came to her hospital room. Today, it's the norm for a baby to be held skin to skin in Labor and Delivery within minutes of the birth, and for those who desire, to be breastfeeding within the hour. But before this norm, I never failed to ask moms about that first hour because early breastfeeding is such a strong predictor of breastfeeding success. In 1993, at the time of Kathy's birth, the rate of initiating breastfeeding within the first hour was a mere 35 percent at our hospital. The norm then was to remove the baby, take him to the nursery, and let the first-year intern complete a newborn exam, honing his/her skills. We are a teaching hospital; of course, interns need opportunities to complete many newborn exams. But now, the exam and all non-emergent care are deferred until the baby has breastfed. Routine vital signs are taken while the baby is skin to skin with his mother. This is true for the bottle-fed babies as well.

This was Kathy's second child, but the first to be delivered at our hospital. Her answer to my question about breastfeeding in Labor and Delivery was gratifying. She said that as staff began to wheel the baby away, the anesthesiologist spoke up on their behalf. Noting how the baby was rooting, he said, "Hold on there, that baby wants to nurse." Even Kathy was moved to have an unexpected advocate. I was thrilled to see the first fruits of staff education paying off. We had a team encircling the mothers, and if one person wasn't conscious about breastfeeding, someone else picked up the slack. It takes a village.

It was many years before we would reach 98 percent of healthy babies, whose moms intend to breastfeed, nursing within the first hour. On a recent Saturday, when I went to see a Hispanic mother who had a cesarean-section, I stopped the nurse in the recovery room to learn that he'd placed the baby skin to skin even before the mother left the operating room. She was nursing upon my arrival. Times have changed.

A study done in the 90s indicated that mothers who were discharged from the hospital early had a better chance to successfully breastfeed than those with a longer stay. It was an obvious indictment on hospital practices at the time. I've been lucky enough to stick around long enough to see those practices change.

The Neighbors' Three Daughters

It is an absolute human certainty that no one can know his own beauty, or perceive a sense of his own worth, until it has been reflected back to him in the mirror of another loving, caring human being.

JOHN J. POWELL

Bernie and Geraldine moved in next door when their girls were still young. When our two girls were middle school-aged, their three girls were frequent playmates. I smile recalling the five girls cheerleading to a sports rally song called the Chase Bugaloo. Two of their daughters occasionally babysat our younger boys when our own girls were unavailable. As early as age 3, my son Andrew would wander away, and Geraldine often answered my worried calls out the front door. "He's over here watching soap operas with me, Chris," she'd say with a broad smile. We lost touch for many years after we moved only a short four blocks away.

A few years later, I encountered Danny, the youngest daughter, on the maternity ward when she was about 22. She was bottle-feeding, but recognizing her name on the census sheet, I stopped in to see her. My visit wasn't about changing her mind about bottle-feeding; it was about renewing a friendship. Did I broach the subject? Of course. But to quote Peggy Robin: *It's wrong for the freedom of one group to turn into the stigmatization of another.* I would never belittle her choice. Just as in her grade school years,

I found her sitting up in bed, sucking her thumb. She stopped long enough to give me a hug and show off her baby.

A few years later, I ran into a grieving Geraldine at the grocery store and was told of Bernie's death from bone cancer. A couple years after this, we met again at the birth of Tenisha's baby. Middle children can be such good caretakers. I learned that Tenisha, always a caring child, had been living with her mom since Bernie's death. She initially wanted to breastfeed, but my efforts to help were unsuccessful and her interest waned. Whether the person is a friend or family member, women make their choices, and we move on. I'm not always privy to how a mom processes the decision to keep trying to nurse, or give it up, but for Tenisha and me, the sun didn't rise and fall on that sole decision. She works at a nearby Target, and we still connect now and then at the store. I see pictures of her growing daughter, and hear updates about her sisters and mom.

Tonya, the oldest, breastfed all her children, though I was only with her after the birth of her last child. Her husband was from Africa, so perhaps he influenced her feeding choice. I often wondered if her early teen exposure to me breastfeeding the boys had anything to do with her choice as well. I wished I'd thought to ask. I had warm relationships with all three girls for 13 years, but Tonya. in particular, perhaps because she was the oldest; or perhaps because she confided in me feeling on the outside of her family because she had a different father and was darker skinned than her sisters. Even with our closeness, there were times when she sneaked into our house while we were all out, just to have something to eat. She had food at home. But we had more options in our pantry and refrigerator.

A year after we moved a few blocks away, Tonya came up to visit and I gave her our rambunctious puppy. She adored Buddy. She wants to one day move her family to Africa. I hope she can.

Conversations Over the Backyard Fence

A thousand threads connect us...and among those fibers, as sympathetic threads, our actions run as causes, and they come back to us as effects.

HERMAN MELVILLE

In 2014, two physicians, both in their first years of fellowships, move in next door. He is an oncologist and rounds both at our hospital and another in the vicinity. She is a psychiatrist. In her fellowship, she works with children. They're easy-going and possess a sweetness I find appealing. Having spent 40 years with physicians-in-training, I have gut feelings about how patients may fare under a given doc. I think both of their patient sets will be glad to have them overseeing their care.

They own two small chunky dogs, Ralph and Izzy. I misunderstood their explanation of how the dogs handle long stretches without their owners at home. Weirdly, I thought she said they wore diapers. I didn't get how that worked, but I know without a doggie door to the fenced backyard, something had to be done.

Ron and I are eating supper on the front porch when we see the two docs walking the dogs, but now there are three. I have a non-rational fear of dogs and would prefer to avoid them, but most Americans love dogs. I'm well aware that I'm in the minority. I get it. In a 2016 Gallup poll, 70% of Americans describe themselves as "dog persons," and 44% own dogs.

We say hello and acknowledge the addition to their family. They begin to laugh.

"Did we tell you we're pregnant?" they ask.

"No! Congratulations!"

"Yeah, we've been trying a while now and just before we got the news, we bought Walter. And we're having twins," they add with irony. They tell us they're due in early Fall.

Indeed, Fall blows in, the leaves on their trees drop, and she delivers. Both babies are discharged with mom. She's told me Halloween is her favorite season, so I buy two small pumpkins, write their names across them, and put them against their front fence, adjacent to the entry. We first see the babies as they come home from their initial pediatric appointment. Mom is making a good supply, but she informs me that they aren't latching very well. They are 4 weeks early, so I am not surprised.

By this time, I have retired from The University of Cincinnati College, which has issued my paychecks for 39 years, and sub-contracted me out to the hospital. I'm sitting in the sun in the backyard writing the poem *Leaves of Absence*, when the new mom comes outside with the three dogs. It's been 4 weeks since I've seen the twins. She's struggling with her supply. It had been so abundant initially, but before they were even 3 weeks old, mom was readmitted for two days for an acute case of gall bladder inflammation.

Over the fence, we chat about ways to increase her milk supply. Still in my chair, I offer ideas using the same casual tone I pick up from mom. She's mildly disappointed, but I sense she'll try what she can and move on if it doesn't work out. If I'd gotten a different vibe, I'd have stood up, gone to the fence to talk, followed up with an email, or checked in with a text to dad three to four days later.

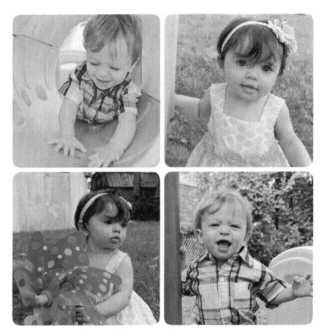

✳ Twins, Charlie, and Sophie ✳

I am not a timid person. I'm fairly assertive, actually, but time in the field has led me to take my cues from the parents. As confident as I am about my knowledge-base, at times I feel a nagging self-doubt about my delivery. Should I have been stronger in the way I made the suggestions, been more proactive to support her, coached her, guided her? However small, it is this little voice that puts me on the fence, and continues to haunt me with the question, "Should I have done more?"

Chapter Sixteen

CLOSE TO HOME
LESSONS FROM MY FAMILY

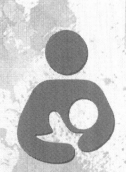

Breastfeeding My Own

---

*No children were harmed or neglected during
the writing of this book.*

ELEANOR ALSPAUGH

My personal experience with breastfeeding was as uneventful as
you can get. No pain, milk came in on time, breastfed four children,
each for 12 to 15 months. There was one small glitch when I went
back to work at 6 months. (Yes! I had a 6-month leave back in 1977.)
I knew I should offer a bottle prior to returning, which I did without
fanfare when Jennifer was baptized at 16-days of age. She took it
easily. "I've got this," I thought.

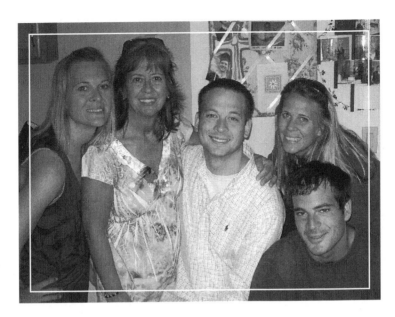

* Amy, Chris, Jason, Jen, Andrew *

Months later, I returned to work. When I got home at midnight from my first evening shift, I crawled in bed and asked Ron, "How'd she do?"

"She didn't," was his casual reply.

"What do you mean she didn't?" I frantically throw my nursing nightgown over my head, waiting for his reply.

"Well, she woke up, I changed the diaper, warmed the bottle, tried to give it to her, and she screamed like a banshee." His eyes are half open as he says this with no emotion.

"And then what?" I am wondering why he seems so relaxed, but I know this is the guy who falls asleep on a dime, so perhaps I should be glad he's talking at all.

"Well, she fell asleep. When she woke up, I changed her diaper, warmed the bottle, and tried to feed her."

"And..."

"And it was the same routine." He's stirring more now, looking a little sheepish, probably wondering what I would have done if the shoe was on the other foot.

"My God, we live 10 minutes from the hospital. Did it not occur to you to bring her up?"

"Hmm, no, not really." Ron is a great entertainer of babies and children. Looking back, I'm sure it was not traumatic for Jen, but I am counting out on my fingers – she went 10 hours with no food. With that, I jump out of bed, skip the diaper change, sit in the rocker, and without her opening those peepers, she is nursing like there's no tomorrow.

"Pleeease, bring her up tomorrow if it happens again."

The next day, she took a bottle as though she'd never resisted.

Trade-Offs

Discernment is a choice between two goods.

THE SPIRITUALITY OF SAINT IGNATIUS

My niece Gina was the first in the next generation of relatives to give birth and Alec breastfed without difficulty. The timing of his birth was ideal for a teacher; six weeks off, return to work six weeks, then summer break. He weaned at close to a year. Annabelle's birth in 2005 was smack in the middle of the school year. With the U.S. policy for maternity leave being far from generous, Gina was back to teaching and her after-school responsibilities in six weeks. Women work valiantly to maintain their milk supplies, but even in the best of circumstances, it's a challenge. September rolled around, and she was faced with the decision of a trade-off – continue to take the extra time to pump at school, or stop pumping and get back to her 9-month-old sooner. This is just one decision of parenthood that can be fraught with emotional landmines for far too many women who are forced to make the choice between two goods.

I thought about Gina 9 years later, when I was developing a PowerPoint presentation for women returning to the workforce. Workforce. The term seems apropos. Most moms report they aren't ready to return to work when their leave is over. Recent legislation made strides to promote pumping in the workplace. Is this doable for all? Apparently, it is for the Pentagon staff. They report that their two pumping rooms are used nearly

700 times per month. There is more work to be done to highlight the benefits to employers so that all women enjoy the support that the military is giving its employees, at least at the Pentagon. In the meantime, my maxim is: make the best choice you can with all the available facts and be at peace with your choice. Gina was. She continued to nurse mornings and evenings through Annabelle's tenth month.

Attachment Parenting

There is no such thing as a baby.
There is only a baby and someone.

DH WINNICOTT

Sharon is Gina's younger sibling by 15 months. She was a happy-go-lucky kid who became a happy-go-lucky adult. The middle-aged, unemployed neighbor who daily jogged our neighborhood, said of her, "When I see Sharon, I always know that there's at least one happy person in the world." He meant it in all sincerity, and he likely needed her wide-smile greetings as his months of job hunting wore on.

Before Sharon became pregnant in 2002, she was working long hours at a local sports bar, and like many of her customers and peers, smoked when she was on break. I was amazed when she told me she stopped smoking cold turkey the day she found out she was pregnant. I considered how I could support her. I thought this would be an upward battle to maintain, and decided I'd stop by her house with a small gift each month and spend a little time with her. At one of those visits, Sharon greeted me wide-eyed at the door, pulling me by the arm into the living room. "You have got to see this, Aunt Chris," she said with enthusiasm. On the television was a segment of a news hour program. It was about attachment parenting. We sat in silence listening together as pediatricians and psychologists explained the philosophy behind the concept. The basic premise is that parents who are attentive to their baby's needs, build trust and security, and security ultimately builds healthy autonomy. In practice, it means holding a newborn skin to skin often, nursing, as well as a belief that a baby's cry is a signal not to be "waited-out," and finally, that close sleep proximity is essential. It also espouses baby-wearing, popularized by the slings and front carriers that were exploding in the first-world market at the time.

When the program ended, Sharon turned to me and declared with determination, "That's the kind of mom I want to be." And indeed, she is. She creates an atmosphere of welcome in her home. It is the gathering place for her adolescent and school-age children and their friends. Sharon provides both structure and fun, a not-so-easy task when managing five between the ages of 7 and 15. I am grateful that for over two years she was the primary caregiver of my own granddaughter, while her parents work.

Parenting philosophies come, and many go. Any of them, though well-intended, can have positive outcomes along with negative consequences. I've never seen any negatives when it comes to Sharon's five children. I'm not fond of the phrase *attachment parenting* because it infers there are many detached parents raising newborns. To be sure, it is not the predecessor of the helicopter parent or the Tiger mom. Still, I think it's important for a mom to think about her philosophy, learn, discuss it with dad and her support system, their care provider, and be open to adapting because life and kids require flexibility. It goes without saying that you can't be someone you're not. Ultimately, parenting styles have to blend with who the mother is, even as parenthood stretches all of us to grow. Having recently read *Bringing up Bebe*, I was keen to learn the interesting parenting philosophy of the French who believe, among other things, that a brief pause, not a mad dash, before picking up a baby upon the first cry, allows them to grow in patience and delayed gratification.

Postscript

Sleep proximity remains a hotly debated topic. It does not inherently mean co-bedding.

In her book, *Parenting without Borders*, Christine Gross-Loh describes solitary sleep as a byproduct of the Industrial Revolution, when living conditions expanded the amount of space available in a home. Soon, separate nurseries were looked at as tangible signs of progress. But around the world, mothers and babies sleeping together remain the norm. When the author spent several years with her family in Japan, she cited one of the most common questions asked of her was, "Is it really true that American parents put their babies to sleep in a separate room?" Yet in Japan, SIDS is quite low, especially when compared to the U.S.

We know from sleep studies, that particularly in the first 6 months, when babies are most vulnerable to sudden infant death, proximity matters. In fact, in 2016 the American Academy of Pediatrics expanded the recommendation to maintain close proximity in the first 6 to 12 months. Bassinettes or pack-and-plays set up in a parent's room are safer for the baby than being in a separate room, where parents strain to hear sounds coming from the nursery. James McKenna, the anthropologist from Notre Dame who studies mother-infant sleep, insightfully reminds us that if anything, parents should be pumping a little sound into the room. We may have the baby monitor backwards. In part, it's deep sleep that puts a baby at risk of SIDS when they could have a short lapse in breathing, with their immature autonomic nervous system responding by "saying" *Breathe*. After returning to the U.S., Gross-Loh's children remarked that they thought the baby monitors they were seeing in many homes were being used for babies to hear their families, not vice versa.

Paternity

With each advancing year, I see fewer pregnant women here in the Midwest wanting to leave home and attend a 90-minute breastfeeding class, let alone a 6-week childbirth series. I attribute this to a combination of factors, including busy working lives and technology's advances that make it more attractive to watch webinars in the privacy of your home at a time convenient for you. When you are confident, have high self-efficacy, and are surrounded by experienced breastfeeding family members, odds are in your favor that you will succeed. Such was the case for my niece, Maria, younger sister to Gina and Sharon. I had her and daddy over in 2013 during the pregnancy, and we sat at the kitchen bar to review a breastfeeding PowerPoint presentation I normally would show to parents in a classroom setting.

The day of the birth, I saw the happy parents in the hospital. Theo was sleeping soundly, having already nursed a few times. We talked about what she and Phil might expect in the coming 24 hours, and I took a few pictures of the family of three. Phil texted a question about poop at about 11 that night, but aside from that, all was well. I'd reminded them earlier that day, tongue-in-cheek, that breastfeeding wasn't rocket science. We are mammals, after all. This little joke wasn't lost on Phil, an aeronautical engineer for General Electric. And while he only had a 3-week paternity leave for Theo, 15 months later, when Cassie came along, it was now up to 6 weeks, which could be taken any time in her first year of life. This is likely the most progressive paternity leave policy for any company in Cincinnati. Should we not feel indignant at the inadequacies of our workplace maternity and paternity leaves? Our country has a long way to go. Kudos to GE.

A Daughter-in-Law
Not Planning to Breastfeed

We cultivate love when we allow our most vulnerable and powerful selves to be deeply seen and known, and when we honor the spiritual connection that grows from that offering with trust, respect, kindness and affection.

BRENE BROWN

AUTHOR

It's tricky to navigate relationships with any in-laws, even when you enjoy their company immensely, the way I do my daughter-in-law, Nicole. She is warm, an attentive listener, and generally says what's on her mind – all traits I appreciate. Still, I suppose I wouldn't talk as freely with her as I would with my own daughters: no holds barred, no filters. Even though I'm pretty transparent, I exercise care when communicating with Nicole, who is married to my youngest son, Jason. Naturally, there isn't the same 29-year history that I have with my son, who likely ignores some of my conversation foibles.

In the course of Nicole's pregnancy in 2013, I sensed breastfeeding wasn't her default option. I gave only tidbits of information now and then, didn't elaborate, just letting them sit in the room between us, as a guest who's quietly in the background. And I told stories of patients I'd seen that day: success stories and success-through-adversity stories. A colleague kindly agreed to stop in at their apartment and talk to Nicole about basic breastfeeding information, and answer any of her concerns or listen to any disinclination to breastfeed that she might feel freer to verbalize to someone other than her mother-in-law.

When I saw her in the recovery room after an emergency cesarean-section, she seemed dazed, as though a whirlwind was happening around her and she was more a spectator than a participant. I've seen this look on other moms when the birth has been emergent. Both parents suddenly have an adrenaline rush with no time to process the facts they are hearing that are leading the doctor to say, "We've got to take her – now." Jason was trying to relay what the obstetrician apparently mentioned in passing at the birth, something about her tongue, when the recovery room nurse interjected, "Oh yeah, the baby's tongue-tied. You'll need that clipped." I was first a grandparent in this situation, not the breastfeeding consultant. I just wanted to see and hold this adorable bundle I saw in mama's arms. Who cares about the skin tag under the tongue? Well, of course I cared. I knew it could impact comfort during feeding, as well as how much milk Abby would be able to obtain. The nursery director arrived, examined the baby and clipped the frenulum, all in fewer than 5 minutes. I know him from rounding on babies where I work. His comment as he exited lets me know that when he'd gotten wind of the tongue-tie, he responded more promptly than was his norm because he recognized the last name. Nicole's mom, Jason, and I were there for the first latch. I suggested she start on the left side first and Abby nursed away.

The post-op meds, the hormones, some soreness with feedings, and I think Nicole and I would agree that those first weeks were not idyllic. By 1 week, she and I took an hour ride north of home to a dentist who used a laser to free the skin tag beneath the upper lip that was unusually attached down to Abby's gums. Even then, it was another week before breastfeeding was comfortable. In classes, I've always told moms that yes, childbirth hurts. Breastfeeding, on the other hand, beyond 10 to 15 seconds of initial discomfort, should not. Many women wouldn't continue to do something 10 times per day that was painful. If that were the case, the human species wouldn't have survived.

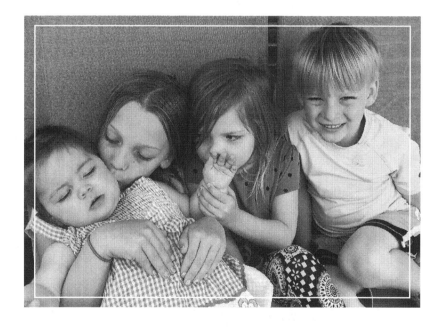

* *Nicole's baby, Olivia Christine with: Ava Rose,*
Abigail Rose, & Nathan James (our grandchildren) *

By 8 weeks, Ms. Abby had a case of colic, that catch-all diagnosis doctors and parents alike use when they don't know why a baby is fussy. Jason and Nicole did a lot of walking the floors in that zombie-like state that parents exhibit when they've been sleep deprived too long. I sympathize with parents up a lot at night. They haven't fully recouped from the prior night and they're back at it for round two, or 22. I am not surprised that sleep deprivation is used as a means of successful interrogation – it's so effective in breaking your spirit.

I recall a conversation with Nicole when Abby was 3 months old. She said that in a moment of frustration, she'd blurted out to Jason, "I wouldn't be doing this if your mom weren't a breastfeeding consultant." And Jas, with his own frustrating sense of powerlessness to help, barked back, "Well quit then. It's nobody's decision, but yours." It was insightful of Nicole, who was still so close to those darker days, to say that wasn't the response she needed from him. She didn't want to quit. She just wanted some measure of compassion. Abby breastfed for a year.

Nicole breastfed Olivia with relative ease, but her second birth had its share of complications that prompted earlier weaning. I care for a super darling granddaughter, prepare her bottles of formula, and feed and care for her three days a week while mommy is at work – and love every minute of it. Did I have an internal struggle when this happened? Of course. Did it last long? Absolutely not. But it resolved when I chose to *love what is*, a philosophy/theology that, I think, has served me well.

It does not escape me that I am a fortunate mother-in-law. Upon my retirement, she wrote:

> *Mom, before I met you, I would have never thought*
> *of breastfeeding my children. It was never even a*

question in my mind, and even leading up to Abby's birth, I was still trying to keep on a brave face, not wanting to disappoint. Luckily, I found that it was an amazing experience, even through all the early struggles, and I would not give back one second of that time with Abby. You gave me that gift!

Nicole

Breastfeeding Sucks, Mom, AND it was Absolutely Wonderful

*Don't get too excited, mom, but I think
I know the meaning of grace. Each night I go
to bed with Ava there in the bassinette next to
me – and I'm afraid to go to sleep. And then
I wake up in the morning, and she's still
breathing. I think that's grace.*

AMY

Amy, my second child, was the third in the extended family to give birth. This happened in 2008 in Columbia, the capital of South Carolina. I remember telling her that she became the mom I always thought she would be. With Ava's birth she seemed, for the first time, at home in her own skin. Though she always intended to breastfeed, she had a bumpy start with nursing that began the day after Ava's birth and persisted for 6 weeks. The day of the birth, there were no nursing issues.

I came into the room the second day and was greeted by a pleasant 6'6" African American gentleman whom Amy introduced as her OB. She hadn't complained about breastfeeding to him. I guess she was waiting to unload her pain on me. Even after the resolution of the first issue, a paper cut-type slice at the base of her nipple, and then later, even after a plugged nipple pore, she was never perfectly comfortable when she breastfed Ava. She attributes that to a painful and persistent forceful let-down of her milk. She's my kid who marches to the beat of a different drum. When she gets a sense of what to do, she's off and running, full speed ahead. Amy grew up to be a strong, kind, and nurturing woman, and a tale of contradictions. She is sensitive, yet bluntly honest, articulate, but sometimes inordinately silent. And like any new mother, hyperattuned to anything that sounds like criticism of this new role she was assuming.

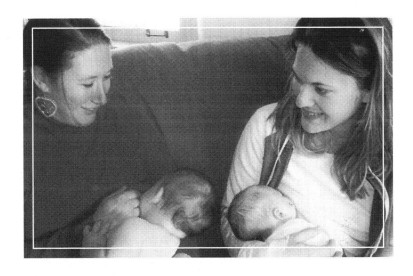

✳ *Cousins Sharon and Amy nursing* ✳

An envelope came in the mail one day. She'd sent her dad and I a photo of Ava, dressed in a plaid outfit, in an infant playground swing, black rubber padding around her chest and between her legs. The moment I slid the picture from the envelope, I was concerned. For a few days, I had it in a frame on the mantle but, not being able to look at it without a sinking feeling, I removed it altogether. Ron didn't see what I saw in that picture, but he trusted my then 16 years of experience in lactation, enough to share in my distress that Ava looked undernourished. Not malnourished, mind you. She just wasn't thriving as I'd expected. But she was smiling, likely at her mother behind the camera, with those sparkly blue eyes that I couldn't see through this black and white glossy. I was sure she had fallen off the growth curve, but it would be another four weeks to verify this at the next doctor appointment. I called Amy before I'd regained objectivity, and that was a mistake. Perhaps it would be more forthcoming to say I called her while my emotions still ran high, and she reacted. She was defensive about her feeding pattern and obviously hurt, interpreting my concern as a challenge to her parenting skills. We went round a few times, getting nowhere, but mutually frustrated. I let it go for the time being, knowing I'd be there in-person in a few weeks and would better understand what was going on.

She was making plenty of milk, so I knew that wasn't part of the problem. Based solely on a gut feeling of how to breastfeed, she was trying to adhere to a feeding schedule for Ava. She had not read, *Babywise*, a popular religious parenting book that advocates not feeding a baby more frequently than every three hours once the baby is all of 3-weeks-old. Some strict followers of this method found themselves in emergency rooms with dehydrated infants, all for lack of feeding them when they showed hunger cues. Years later, even that author admitted that all babies are different. Amy tells me now the idea of a schedule was mostly attributed to wanting to avoid the pain of every feeding. When I wasn't in the same city readily available to observe and support, and I couldn't get the full picture over the phone, it wasn't easy to fully appreciate what in the world was going on in South Carolina.

It is a dance I do when I tell any parent *trust yourself*, because in fact, this has to be tempered with some information or experience, which most first-time parents don't have. Guidance is warranted. It just gets more complicated when it's your daughter. When Ava would fuss, if it was less than three hours since the previous feeding, Amy would swing with her, dance with her, anything to quiet her. And in fact, Ava often quieted, which further justified Amy's assumption that it couldn't be hunger. My thoughts needlessly ran to extremes. I thought about the stages of Trust vs Mistrust, and the virtue of Hope, about which the developmental psychologist, Erik Erikson wrote.

I waited anxiously for that next pediatrician's appointment. It was hard being 500 miles away. And more difficult still to know that I had taught every pediatric intern in the city, given a monthly lecture on breastfeeding management, and yet had no influence on my daughter's situation. Her husband could see our conversations only upset Amy, and he was equally defensive. Amy called to report the weight. It sounded like the doctor was very sensitive and non-alarmist, telling her that a slight alteration in feeding pattern would bring Ava right back up to her normal growth curve. Amy was eagerly compliant and fed her more frequently. It took a stranger, albeit one with authority in the matter.

Even then, I could barely wait for the bimonthly check-ups to learn of her weight progression. Amy came to both dread and resent it. I wish I could have handled it all differently, and when Nate was born two-and-a-half years later, we never spoke of weights, nor did we need to. He breastfed without difficulty. When Amy learned I was repeating her phrase, "Breastfeeding Sucks Mom" during the monthly resident lecture, she requested I at least add that it was absolutely wonderful too.

How Do I Love Thee,
Let Me Count the Blades

What Spouses Endure

Love is an Intention and an Action.

SCOTT PECK

Ron and I have several important values in common. We believe in being mindful of a spiritual journey on a daily basis. We believe that we have responsibilities beyond ourselves, and toward the common good. We have a dominant Mother/Father archetype, which bond us together as we purposefully consider the needs of our four adult children and their mates. We believe in a strong work ethic, which means you give 100 percent when you're on the job.

The problem is how I lived out this last value. First, I had an illusion that if I just stayed longer at work, I'd be ahead of the game the following day. Second, I have trouble with time management. For Ron, time management is second nature. He can look at his tasks for the day, prioritize, and understand how much time he can devote to each, and arrive home on time for dinner. In the time management world of Stephen Covey, I tend to assess many things as both Urgent and Important. Herein lies the problem. I can look at my tasks for the day, prioritize, and then allow any number of those tasks to spill over into the next task's time slot. I rarely make it home for dinner on time.

I feel bad for Ron; but as he's said many times, this does no good. As unintentional as my behavior has been, it has made him feel like he plays second fiddle to my career. I start the day with the best intention of leaving work on time ... and what? What happens? I might see that a patient has delivered whom I'd taught in class, and know that she'll appreciate my stopping in, if only briefly. I may overhear a staff member giving inaccurate information and feel compelled to take 10 minutes at the end of the day to talk to her since I likely won't get a chance the next day.

Some of my colleagues might skip the patient who has been using formula all night, but I have a drive to understand what happened. If she just wanted to switch feeding methods, fine, but sometimes she has something going on that will go unaddressed if someone doesn't stop in to see her. In such situations, a day of giving formula can turn into a whole year. It may be a mother who's had a radiographic scan who thinks breastfeeding is now prohibited. It might be a mother who has gotten sore and needs assistance, or warms to the idea of a 12-hour break from nursing, instead of totally switching to formula. Perhaps I see the phone lit up with a voice-mail message and feel that if it's a patient's urgent need, she shouldn't have to wait another 16 hours for a response. The list is endless. A friend once said that I'm responsible to a fault, and that was not a compliment. To be honest, when it comes to phone calls, I have often made them as I drove home, just to save time.

Still, I was late at least 80 percent of the time, mostly because I put too many things into the Urgent and Important quadrant, and I left Ron out of that quadrant. Usually, I was an hour to an hour-and-a-half late. Worse yet, I'd often forget to call, or I'd call as I was driving home, which he considered a waste. If I'd have just called at 5 o'clock, he'd have known to prepare and eat dinner without me. It was never the cooking he minded; it was the dinners well past a reasonable hour that would get to him. By and large, he eventually gave up on me ever getting home on time. But then there would be the morning promises, "I'm in the NICU today; it'll be easy to leave at 5." Or, "The census is low; it'll be easy to leave at 5." Or, "I'm going in early; I'll be home by 4." Even the latter, he quit believing. He just said that those were the days I worked at least an hour longer. That is not to say he couldn't roll his eyes at me and still joke about it. That happened some of the time. But we are talking about a long career, and the patience of even a most forgiving man can run thin.

Such was the case on a particular August evening. This was 37 years into our marriage and 20 years in the lactation field. I'd told him in the morning that I was going to work a little later in the office after seeing patients because I needed to sift through some data for a publication I was working on.

I had a heavy load of patients that day, and didn't begin to make my way over to the NICU office until after 6. Once I was in the doors of the NICU, a nurse stopped to ask me to co-check milk coming from the freezer and going home with a mom and baby that evening. Then a mother saw me when she was signing in at the front desk and asked to speak a few moments. By 6:30, I was in the office and rolling up my sleeves for the work ahead. I needed to review data located in three different places, and confirm that all the numbers matched so that the data could be included in a publication. It was a year's worth of information and tedious work, and I called home to tell Ron I'd be later than

I first thought, "likely not until 9," I said, in response to his question about when I'd arrive home. He was very understanding and was already in process of preparing dinner.

I was on a roll and excited to see the actual numbers lining up. Four hours later, I took a stretch break. Seeing it was nearly 11, I decided not to call, since he'd already be in bed. I had said I'd be late, after all. The work was complete around 1:30 a.m. After emailing the doctor who was spearheading the publication, I exited the stairs and went out through the emergency room, a security guard escorting me to the car. I left tired, but felt some exhilarated with a great sense of accomplishment.

Arriving home at 2 in the morning, I entered the bedroom. Ron wasn't there. I didn't bother to look for him, thinking that he was sleeping on the floor of another bedroom, something he'd do sometimes when his back was bothering him. The next morning, he was already outside working on his car when I stepped out the door at 7:45 to leave for another day's work.

"What happened to you last night?" I queried innocently.

"What happened to me? What happened to you?" Uh-oh. I recognize that tone of voice. I'm in trouble and I can feel my heart pick up its pace.

"What? I told you I was working late." I'm fumbling with the keys now, even as I fumble for the right answers.

"You said 9 o'clock." His voice is staccato and he's not making eye contact as he polishes the wheel rims.

"Yeah, I know, but time got away from me, and when I was going to call again, I knew you'd already be in bed." It seemed like an honest and legitimate response, but a voice in my head is asking me whether I'll ever learn.

"Well, I slept with my phone right at the bedside."

"Well, why didn't you call?" How could this not be a reasonable question? But he stops now and glares.

"Why didn't *you* call?" he shot back, but I'd already explained that and figured it was rhetorical.

"I had *no* idea what you were doing or who you were with," he went on.

"But I told you what I was doing. I'm sorry. Really."

It was then I realized he actually doubted my story. I eyed my watch and accepted I'd be late for work. Returning to the house, I sat down in front of the computer and went into my work email. Thank God I had emailed Laura right before I'd left work. She was the lead physician preparing the manuscript, and she was a she, which suddenly seemed an important detail. I printed the email and tried to give it to him, but he was in no mood for explanations or justifications. When I left for work, we were disconnected.

I made sure I was home on time that day. As I drove up to the house, I noticed miniature American flags placed all over the front and side yards. "What's he up to?" I wondered briefly. Minutes later, Ron was coming out the front door as I was going in. I began again with a sincere apology. He cut me off. "I'm not interested in an apology; I'm interested in a change of behavior."

Yikes. Things were no better. Even then I was mentally rationalizing and dismissing the problem thinking, "What is the likelihood that I'd ever need to do data collection like that again before retirement?"

Realizing I wasn't going to change Ron's mood, I went inside and changed into running clothes. As I headed down the driveway, he came around the side of the garage.

"Whoa, wait a minute. Where are you going?" It was obvious. I take to the park most summer evenings for a walk or run. He pointed to the American flags.

"See those flags in the yard?" Yes, of course I do, I thought, but I knew better than to speak.

"I want you to pull up all the bent grass you see in each area." Bent grass was the latest weed we were fighting in a large and otherwise lovely yard. I felt like a school child being assigned a punishment, but dutifully knelt and began the task. He walked away to his own work in the backyard.

I was on my knees for well over an hour when he came back into the front yard holding his cellphone.

"It's Jason. He wants me to put you on speaker." Our son Jason had just turned 25, and was hiking in the Smokey Mountains with his girlfriend.

"Wanted you to know I just proposed to Nicole, and she said yes," he said excitedly.

Life and mood can change on a dime. Ron and I listened to every wonderful and funny detail of his story, and made plans to celebrate when they returned home. The air lifted between us and we were reconnected.

Three years later, at our 40th wedding anniversary, Ron's speech to guests mentioned that one of the things he loves about me is my love for the moms in my care.

Some would say this is a story about role reversal, husband complaining about the wife's work schedule and her passion about her career. Perhaps so. Many laugh when I repeat the part about the American flags and the bent grass. It's funny, I

know, and I still smile at the scene. But I am remembering how
I was loved enough to be worried about by a man who wanted
and deserved the same love and consideration in return.

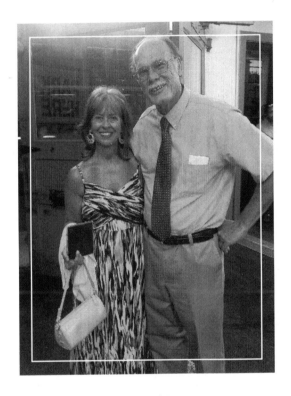

✳ Chris and Ron ✳

Chapter Seventeen

SOCIAL MEDIA, INSTANT MESSAGING, SKYPE, CALLS, ADOPTION, AND HEALTH FAIRS

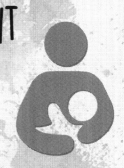

OTHER ENCOUNTERS

Instant Messaging

Let us swim together in the ocean of our being.

JONATHAN LOCKWOOD HUIE

I see her husband's Facebook post and realize my young friend has had an emergency C-section eight weeks prior to her due date. I'm horrified as I read the life-threatening circumstances surrounding the birth. I'd messaged Alaina via Facebook, a couple weeks prior to see how the pregnancy was coming along and if, like her oldest sister, she'd be delivering at UCMC. She replied that she was going to travel 45 minutes north and under a midwife's care, have a hospital-based water birth. (This method of birthing was made famous in the 70s by the French obstetrician, Fredrick Leboyer in his book, *Birth Without Violence*). Water birth yes, 45-minute drive north with a second pregnancy–I was worried. I spoke my cautions and wished her well. Alaina knew I was available if there were any breastfeeding concerns, but I replied to Steve's post with the offer of help if needed.

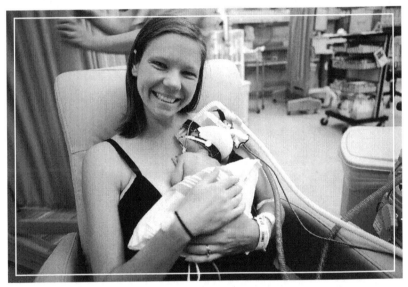

Alaina skin to skin with her darling daughter, Poppy. *

I describe Alaina to others as the same smiley-faced adult as the 5-year-old at the bus stop headed to school with my boys. This went on for six years. She's a gem. I instant message her later that day to check in. How was her blood count? Did she get transfused in a timely manner? How much milk was she making? I suggested she ask her delivering hospital if they had the video, *A Preemie Needs His Mom*. It's super helpful, having 4, 15-minute segments, covering: Benefits of Human Milk and Kangaroo Care, Strategies to Build a Supply, and Direct Breastfeeding a Preemie. I tell Alaina what she might ask for regarding advancing breastfeeding and give her a timetable for when the baby might be ready, and offer to come up to her hospital if she needs assistance or an advocate. From her response, I learn that the baby was transported to our NICU shortly after the birth. She and her baby are in excellent hands.

We messaged the next day and again five days later. I also let the nutritionist and NICU lactation consultant know of our friendship. A week after our first contact, Poppy is off of the CPAP breathing apparatus and I come into the unit long enough to help Alaina breastfeed her daughter. They do beautifully. Mommy is a fatigued bundle of joy and making 32 ounces per day! I tell her this is quite a feat at day 10 for a mom who'd had a placental abruption.

"At home, I pump while watching Poppy on the BabyCam. I think it really helps me. I'm so glad the NICU offers this service. Even out of town family can see her once I give them the code."

And as she tells me more details surrounding the birth, I am quietly saying, *Thanks be to God.* You don't pass out a mile from the hospital, expel placental fragments in the car and come out all right. In fact, she said the surgeon told her later that another 10 minutes and they would have lost both of them. What a sea change that 10 minutes made.

Poppy will be nursing a couple times a day for now. We make plans for another latch when I'm scheduled to work two days later. In the meantime, Laia, our NICU LC will be available to her.

I am amazed and grateful for the gift of social media when it's used to stay connected to people you care about.

The Prisoner

We learn from the gardens to
deal with the most urgent question of
the time: How much is enough?

WENDELL BERRY

A few moms have, sadly, been incarcerated just prior to delivery. Someone or an entity is given at least short-term custody of the baby, and the mother is returned to complete her incarceration. In these situations, it's been entirely left up to the jail staff whether she can use the hand pump she's been given, and whether they are willing to store the milk for family to retrieve every day or two. But the prisoner that had me most concerned one Saturday afternoon was the mother of a 3-and-a-half year-old who called and began the conversation with, *I feel like I'm a prisoner of my daughter.*

She went on to explain how the child sleeps between mom and dad each night, and does 90 percent of her nursing at night. Awakening every couple hours, mom is exhausted. As she continued, I could hear her beginning to talk herself out of the notion of weaning, feeling that she is still offering immunization through her milk. Then she would slip back into a litany of how it was taking a toll on her. Her vacillating spoke volumes of the dilemma of competing values she was grappling with.

After intermittent questions to understand the family system better, I offered, "the operative word here seems to be prisoner." That opened a flood-gate of tears. Usually I find moms just need a sounding board as they navigate the poorly lit path of parental decisions. Typically, they get themselves to the clearing of their own devices.

By the end of the conversation, she had decided to talk to her mom about keeping her daughter for a weekend. Grandmas can be good distractors. Complimenting her on the idea, I asked her to call me back if that didn't do the trick. I never heard back. I hoped that was a good sign, but it was no guarantee.

Many professionals recommend baby-led weaning, but we have to remember this is a dance between two, and as a lapel button given me by a midwife says, it's imperative to *Listen to Women.*

The First Ladies' Health Fair

Invisible threads are the strongest ties.

FRIEDRICH NIETZSCHE

It was a warm Sunday afternoon when I volunteered to staff the UC Reproductive Health booth at the First Ladies' Health Initiative. This was one of 30 fairs at Black churches across the city aimed at reducing the disparity in health between the African American and other races. It was the brainchild of the mayor's wife and a cluster of First Ladies, the pastor's wives, and women in leadership in Black churches.

The church and neighborhood were familiar. Mother of Christ, in Winton Terrace, is our sister parish, and this is the neighborhood where for five years I'd gone to various apartments on behalf of St. Vincent de Paul, whose mission is to meet concrete needs like food, kitchen equipment, clothes, gas bills, and summer fans—and less concrete, prayer needs. We are in the trenches with the clients. We can't avoid it. But today was about information.

Familiarizing myself with the literature, I spread it across the round table bedecked in its blue plastic tablecloth. It included titles like Becoming a Dad, Planning Pregnancy After a Premature Birth, Healthy Eating, Creating a Dream for your Life, The Top 10 Reasons to Breastfeed, Building a Milk Supply, and Healthy Relationships. This latter was code for identifying and fleeing abusive relationships.

The head of the parish food pantry had donated 32 boxes of organic baby food due to expire in 20 days. In each box were eight squeezable containers. Most 8-month-olds would be delighted to suck on these combos that included foods, such as rice, applesauce, carrots, and squash. These colorful, wouldbe attention-grabbers, lure people to my table out of curiosity. Across the way, Children's Hospital employees are very busy with immunizations, flu shots, and school physicals.

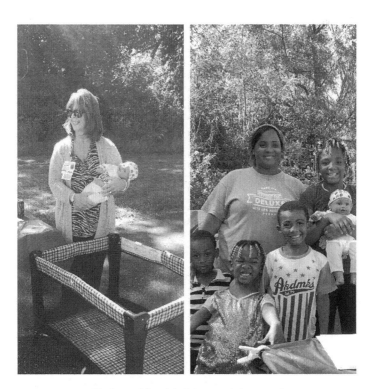

Chris and health fair participant who breastfed her four happy children

The onslaught of mothers, children, grandmothers, and great-grandmothers was astounding. I expected 10 to 20 at most. There were well over 100. Few men were present. I counted less than 10 over the four hours, and only two to three who appeared to be less than 30 years old. To be fair, it was at the exact time of the Bengals-Seahawks football game, but I doubt that even a bye-week would have yielded different results. Where are the men? Not at the fair, few in this church, and few on the maternity ward after a birth. I cannot let my mind go there because the issues are so complex and well beyond my sphere of influence. But I do know that the state of Ohio is the only state on the books to have a Commission on Fatherhood. I met the wonderful gentleman who heads up the program in Hamilton County, where 1,000 dads are mentored each year. Some of their programs include Breast for Success, On My Shoulders, Love Notes, and Father Factors. They are doing a great job.

The fair became an opportunity to plant small seeds, affirm, and listen. The younger ones come with children or girlfriends. There are only seconds to assess and anticipate what topics were pertinent for their needs. Do you have children? Tell me their ages? Do you plan to have more? Have you ever had a preemie? How did you feed your babies? I was surprised how many at least partially breastfed. Why do I find this significant? It's not because of the outcomes of a healthier baby. With limited support systems, few role models, and pressure to do otherwise, they chose the feeding method that required their sole presence. I am praying quietly that this attachment connection will carry the child a little further down the road of the American dream. I am hoping that this decision reflects a spark of determination in their mothers that will carry them down this same road.

The sun touched my back, warming me all day. As the conversations continued through the afternoon, I was touched in that soul-connecting way genuine encounters provide. I ran out of give-away bags an hour before the event was over, but no one seemed to care. They had things on their mind they were spreading across this table of comradery. We only scratched the surface. I wished I was more adept at helping them unpack their stories.

In the hospital, I am used to narrowing the conversations to stay far from the neighborhoods and lives to which these mothers will be returning. In my work setting, I am warm and well-received. I wonder if we both know we are avoiding more dire topics, me in my lab coat and them in their hospital gown, sterile and removed from home. Maybe it's a blessing. I don't know if I could do the job of breastfeeding support while wearing my heart on my sleeve. But today seems full of hope and promise and being gathered as we were in a church parking lot seems perfectly natural.

The Mother in Ecuador

Sometimes reaching out and taking someone's hand is the beginning of a journey.

VERA NAZARIAN

Valerie emailed me, asking if I'd be open to helping Jane with a breastfeeding issue. Jane's email address was included. Of course, I would. I've had my daughter's high school friend over when she'd had problems with her first. I'd had my son's high school buddy over with his wife when she was struggling early on. So, why not? It's not uncommon for friends or family to call Ron for advice about remodeling. It's what we do. However, Jane lives in Ecuador, and while we initially emailed so I could get the back-story, we Skyped so we could talk face-to-face.

I hadn't seen Jane since she was in high school. She's now 33. She didn't run with my kids, but Amy had spent some time with her when she agreed to chaperone a group of high school students on a protest bus trip down to Georgia's School of the Americas. The protests lasted over ten years, until in 2000, the academy began to require a minimum of eight hours of classes on human rights. I simply remember Amy coming home and declaring, "That Janie Becker, and her buddy Laura, are radicals." (Laura now lives in Thailand, where she gave birth within a few months of Jane.)

She writes me the backstory with the details I need to understand her situation, sends a video so I can see how

Victoria acts at the breast, and we Skype a few days later. Jane is on her couch, and I have to comment that looking at the background of her apartment, I'd have thought she was in the U.S. It seems modern, carpeted, with furniture that could have come from Ikea. I'm so naïve. I presumed she was in some bush country, or trying to save the country's rainforest from first-world corporations. She laughs. She is there because her husband works for his father's business. It's about family. Talking to Jane feels like talking with her mom, Ann. There is a comfort level of familiarity because we have some common ground, though Jane and I are 30 years apart in age.

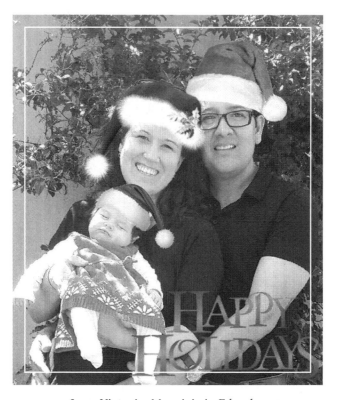

✳ Jane, Victoria, Mauricio in Eduador ✳

She tells me she's "self-diagnosed," and it's an oversupply issue. Victoria begins to feed, fusses unhappily, and comes off the breast. She goes on and off and on and off until finally settling into nursing, eats for 30 minutes each side, then falls asleep. The bad feedings are short and interspersed with screams. For Victoria to stay asleep, Jane holds her in her arms. While she loves this baby she birthed naturally in water five weeks prior, she'd like to lay her down and nap herself, or get something else productive done. This is frustrating, of course. We put our heads together and strategize and come up with a plan. Her husband, Mauricio, comes in before we say goodbye, and I get to meet him "in person."

We keep in touch through several emails. Victoria is crying less and sleeping for longer intervals now, and so is Jane. She has bought a swing that in the U.S. would cost $80, but in Ecuador, was $240. This cost makes no sense when so many things are so darn inexpensive there. Why this? She knows I'm available to Skype again if needed. I tell her I really want to stay in a Spanish-speaking country for a few months to improve my language skills, and she welcomes me to Ecuador. This age of technology has its downside, but for what Jane needed, it is a good thing—wonderful even. Much more important than our time together is the time Victoria's Cincinnati grandparents can spend with their family.

Bearing and Raising Children

Adoption

Instead of growing in my belly,
they grew in my heart.

ANONYMOUS

＊

Stacie, the NICU nutritionist, and human-milk proponent extraordinaire, stops me when I'm walking through the crowd of providers as they begin morning rounds. They're in the corridor outside the pods this morning, discussing something particularly confidential before beginning in Pod A.

"Did you know the Monet baby is getting all human milk?" she asks with a look of incredulity. I don't recognize the name, and by the blank look I must have on my face, she goes on to explain.

"The baby's up for adoption. Ah, and there's the adoptive mother scrubbing in now. You better speak to her. Let me know what's going on."

"Good morning," I greet her and the presumptive adoptive father. "You two are up bright and early!" I say as the parents are both dutifully using the plastic picks to clean under their nails after they scrub in. "My name's Chris, I'm the lactation consultant for the NICU."

As she dries her hands, she extends her right hand in introduction. "My name's Shelly. I know, it's super early for us, too, but Camille was low on breast milk when we left last night, so I wanted to get milk here before her nine o'clock feeding.

"Yes, the nutritionist just told me she's gotten all milk since her admission. Are you lactating for another child as well?"

"No, I've been pumping for 2 months and taking fenugreek and blessed thistle. I began when I knew the birth was getting close, and started making substantial amounts of milk a few weeks ago. I did this for Kylie, our other adopted child, but actually, I'm getting more milk this time."

When I ask if she'd given birth to other children, she replies she has. "Yes, two. I think that's why this works so well—at least that's what I've read."

"You're right. Nice job. Have you breastfed Camille yet?"

"I began a couple days ago, when the docs said she'd likely be going home today." We're thrilled—she's only 3 weeks, you know. I called in today. The nurse says she's over 4 pounds!"

"Once you get to the bedside, I'd like to give you a guideline about how to proceed with advancing more breastfeeding. Sound good?"

I return to Stacie and let her know the story. Together, we're amazed. I don't know the odds for making milk in a situation like this, but I do know that people often surprise me with their success against those odds.

✳✳

You don't have to give birth to
someone to have a family.
We're all family—extended family.

SANDRA BULLOCK

There were other adoptive parents I worked with. A gay couple from the west side of town arranged an open adoption with a young woman from Pleasant Ridge, a central suburb in Cincinnati. I helped her establish her supply with a pump. The dads planned to make a daily trip to Pleasant Ridge to pick up milk for their son. They had a plan, and it worked for at least the months the birth-mom kept up with me, calling with questions from supply to medications.

The Golden Ticket

*When a woman is talking to you, listen to
what she says with her eyes.*

VICTOR HUGO

For all the benefits of breastfeeding, it is no panacea. Breastfed children do get sick. It's a harsh reality, especially when it's a critically ill child. And while breastfeeding lowers the risk of pre-menopausal breast cancer, ovarian cancer, osteoporosis, stroke, and heart disease, women who have breastfed also get sick.

When I saw that our Barrett Cancer Treatment Center was sponsoring a free community-wide education symposium, I approached the organizers to see if I could submit a poster. The idea was received with enthusiasm, and I was there all day, manning the table one Saturday in 1998.

It was a slow, but steady stream from 10 in the morning to 4 in the afternoon. The men glanced at the poster and wandered by. The women, and they were the majority, were more likely to stop and read. I passed out informative literature, some to women clearly childbearing age, and many to women who said they planned to pass it along to their daughters or granddaughters. Those who had breastfed spoke positively about the experience, seeming to be happy to be diverted from the gloomy world of cancer information. Some women complained that they breastfed successfully without the ton of support they saw surrounding their birthing daughters; bad for those women, but good news for their daughters.

Two separate conversations stay with me, even now. They were nearly identical. The grandmotherly woman began, "It didn't work for me." The middle-aged woman, "It didn't work for my daughter."

"I am so sorry," I begin, and remain quiet several moments as they take their time deciding whether to tell their story to a perfect stranger. I mourn with them, empathize, touch their shoulders, sigh. There are no tears, only sad eyes, as their realities sit between us like a bump on a log, only it's a lump on the breast that each of them are discussing in a voice of resignation.

Although I explain to each how much I wish breastfeeding were a total preventive tool in the arsenal against cancer, I tell them how I hate that these huge population-based studies can't predict what will happen to an individual woman, me, them, their daughters. Life is unfair. They seem to appreciate the frustration in my voice. And it is real. How I wish I had the Golden Ticket.

Follow-Up Calls

*Don't waste your time dividing the world
into the good guys and the bad guys. Hold
them both together in your own soul—where
they are anyway—and you will have held
together the whole world. You will have
overcome the great divide in one place of
spacious compassion.*

RICHARD ROHR

OFM

The sun glistens on the red and white flowers as I enter the courtyard. This is my favorite spot. Each May, there's a huge tent set up as we celebrate Hospital Week with a picnic. The food is served by the chief nursing officer and other upper-management celebrities. Even among staff, there is beautiful diversity and it's captured in a mosaic of our photos displayed in the lobby. The digital image it creates is a photo of the front of the hospital and beneath, it read: 5,000+ staff of University Hospital Welcomes You.

Today, the noise of the helicopter's blades beat a rhythmic thump, thump, thump above me. There are residents in blue scrubs chatting on a nearby bench. They raise their voices above the din, and I hear them chiding the young female physician among them about the colored tattoo visible below her short-sleeved scrub top. A gentleman visitor is writing notes in what appears to be a journal as he sits on the bench adjacent to the hospital entrance. There is something so comforting about the familiarity of my surroundings, even though the characters in the scene change from day to day.

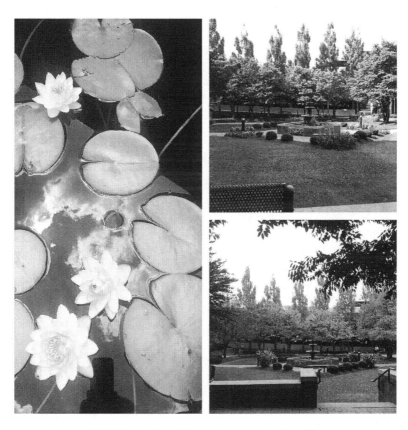

∗ UCMC courtyard in every season of my life ∗

On another square wood bench, two women in scrubs are talking. A wide-lettered "RN" hangs below their photo ID's. I ask, "Do you mind?" pointing toward the bench and they reply in a welcoming manner. I sit to read the text sent by Jen, my oldest. She's in Belgium for a conference where she's giving a presentation on chaos theory. I've asked what that means so many times it's embarrassing, but Jen dutifully gives her explanation to the layperson I am, in simple descriptors that a seasoned PhD can capably provide. It's above me. I wonder about things like, what exactly is a Tootsie Roll? Or the existential question of *Why*. I'm realizing we have our own version of chaos as I overhear one nurse tell the other about the in-service she'd just attended on what to do in the event of a confrontation with an *active shooter*. In my 40 years here, I've never heard of this being an issue at our hospital, but as the nurse repeats some of the information she's been given, I learn that our emergency department, housed adjacent to this picturesque courtyard, treats over 50 gunshot wounds each month. It's shocking news. For a while, it had gotten better in Cincinnati. When these numbers last peaked, the physician overseeing the ER met with city council members to discuss guns fatalities and injuries, and efforts were made to remedy the crisis. Now, as I hear the helicopter's engine, my mind flashes to a MASH unit because we're in a quasi-war zone of our own in this city and country. It's disquieting.

Situated now at the desk, I pull up the Excel spread sheet with the list of the month's discharges, and begin to jot down the mothers' names and their birth dates. From there, I open the electronic medical record to the *Snapshot* section. It tells me each mother's preferred language. English, of course, Spanish, French, Oromo, Cantonese, Arabic, Fulani, Amharic, Farsi, Bambara, Soninke, Nepali, and Tigrinya. It's going to be a cumbersome set of phone calls requiring me to use an interpreter for over half of the 22 calls I'll make today. Some of the African languages are so infrequent that even the *Pacific Interpreters* agency subcontracts out, and one lingers on the other end of the line while they find someone available. All but one of the interpreters is male today, and I wonder what they think of these breast, babies, and breastfeeding conversations. It's a joy, actually, and I love the diversity and am so happy we have a way to follow-up on all breastfeeders, not just the English-speaking moms.

Before I leave, the attending pediatrician asks me to see the mom in room 3362. During the pregnancy, it was identified that her baby had Trisomy 13. This is quite different than Down's syndrome, which is Trisomy 21. Trisomy 13 is usually not compatible with life, and I ask Dr. Jenny if there's a chance of a misdiagnosis.

"Perhaps," she says, "we've sent off DNA." She continues, "I tried to latch the baby on, but she didn't sustain a suck. I don't know if she was just not ready to eat or if she needed the help of a nipple shield." Jenny is a hands-on attending. The patients love her, and we're thrilled that she planned to sit for her lactation board exam in July 2017.

I'm sensitive to the fact that the mother may be feeling stressed and enter the room greeting everyone with a pleasant tone. "My name's Chris. I'm the breastfeeding consultant. The pediatrician has asked me to check in on you." Mom greets me and welcomes me warmly into the room.

"I remember you! You helped me with my first baby."

"Mama," she says to the older woman in the room, "she taught my breastfeeding class."

"So, you've breastfed before, huh?"

"All three for a year each!" She can see I'm quite impressed, and I tell her that if she were feeling better, I'd have her help me round on the other moms, and this makes her smile.

"Do you have a picture of your first?" I ask. And she flips open her phone and shows me a handsome young man in a white shirt and tie. "How old is he?"

"Seventeen. And yeah, know, you gave me a *Boppy* for attending the class." She proceeds to repeat a couple things I said in class and they sound exactly like something I'd say.

"Wow. Your memory is blowing my mind."

We don't talk about the diagnosis. She proceeds to latch the baby "the way I taught her," which she says was different than the pediatrician who'd been in to see her. The baby nurses well for 10 minutes. It'll be a few days before we understand if her daughter is able to effectively breastfeed and grow because as mom knows, it'll be better for the baby's brain development. Dad comes in during the feeding, and I emphasize that both of them should be holding their daughter skin to skin to further help in brain development, and they nod in agreement.

It's quiet when I re-enter the courtyard to leave for the day, except for the thump, thump, thump of my full heart.

Military Wives

Special Forces

Victor Frankl wrote that human beings create meaning in three ways; through their work, through their relationships, and by how they choose to meet unavoidable suffering. Every life brings hardship and trial, and every life also offers deep possibilities for meaningful work and love ... I've learned that courage and compassion are two sides of the same coin.

ERIC GREITENS

THE WARRIOR'S HEART

I've wondered at times, if the difficult circumstances many women experience surrounding birth piques a special force within them to endure and come out a wiser, more compassionate person. For me, it's so very different being with mothers and fathers who can leisurely take in the excitement of new parenthood compared to those who have a brief leave from deployment, or are on the verge of deployment. It was bittersweet when one of the mothers got to see her deployed husband mid-deployment for two weeks, coinciding with an induced labor to assure his presence. These are people who know there is no promise of tomorrow. Other mothers say goodbye for a year within weeks of the birth. Such was the case of my own daughter after their second was born. I wouldn't wish that on anyone, but military decisions aren't based on a grandmother's wishes.

When I had a Skype session with a wife of a Special Forces operative, he was between missions and home for the birth. Once discharged from the hospital, this mom couldn't find a breastfeeding consultant that could solve the feeding issues confronting her. She began pumping milk while she and her baby tried to make a go of nursing. If you are wondering, yes, it's nearly impossible to understand, let alone assist, in problem-solving via Skype, but it is an avenue for encouraging moms and exploring ideas that could address concerns. It's also a way to provide tips to build a milk supply and occasionally, to identifying the source of blatant problems.

While Vinnie never latched, she was undeterred when attempting with her second, who nursed for a year. I'm encouraged when Kelly, like so many women, can come to peace about the outcome of one breastfeeding experience, yet re-enter that arena a few years later with even stronger resolve. Of course, this is a dance. There are two partners, so even the most determined of mothers do not always get the outcome they so very much desire.

With her third baby, Kelly was back to pumping due to pain with latch. She knew it wasn't normal. This time, she understood why. A week after his birth, she texted me a picture of her son's mouth. Within two days, she had an appointment with a pediatric ear, nose, and throat specialist (ENT) for evaluating the skin tag under the tongue. Commonly referred to as tongue-tie, this short frenulum can cause poor weight gain as well as soreness. In the best-case scenario, the physician will understand her concern and appreciate that the function of the tongue was hampered by how tightly tethered the frenulum was to the floor of the mouth. One would never guess that a millimeter could matter—

except for a Special Forces sharp shooter, I suppose. Last report, his tongue was more mobile after the small scissor snip of the skin tag, he was latching again, and she wasn't in horrendous pain. Her final text: *Things are going sooo much better now.*

It takes a warrior's heart to overcome obstacles like Kelly has had in nursing and in life. She and Tommy are suited for each other. They both have had their missions. Over their married years, he's been deployed three times with several extended absences for training. We have gotten better as a nation in recognizing the service of our armed forces. I don't think we express as often as we should that a grateful nation honors the family's sacrifice. We do.

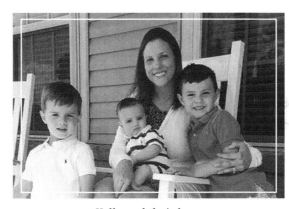

✳ *Kelly and their boys* ✳

Chapter Eighteen

SHIPPING OUT

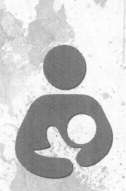

The Gift

Even after all this time
the sun never says to the earth,
"You owe me."
Look what happens with a love like that,
It lights the whole sky.

HAFIZ

Military personnel aren't all that's being shipped out. In the past 20 years, I've worked with mothers who have shipped over 1,500 ounces of their milk to milk banks in Denver, Colorado and Columbus, Ohio. All milk came from mothers pumping for preemies in the NICU. For some, it was because they had an overabundant supply and felt donating the milk was a way of giving to other babies whose mothers struggled with supply. For a few, it was because their tiny baby did not survive, and they wanted him or her to have a legacy. Some said that stopping the pumping process confronted them with their loss, but gradually letting go of pumping was a gentler way through their grieving process. I could only support them and encourage them to trust themselves. They'd know when it was right to stop. One mom with a surviving twin felt her body still thought she had two babies to feed. I would describe each of them as generous and courageous women.

As of mid-2017, there are 22 milk banks in the U.S. under the auspices of the non-profit, Human Milk Banking Association of North America, and additional sites in Canada. A report from 2014 indicates that over 3.7 million ounces were distributed that year alone. Most of the recipients were babies in newborn intensive care units. The mothers who donate milk must complete a written health screen and blood screens, and have their doctor and their baby's doctor sign-off in approval. They are not paid. Milk is then sterilized by pasteurization and re-examined for bacteria. In February 2016, as the water crisis in Flint, Michigan unfolded, the milk bank issued a statement calling for access to donor milk for mothers whose lead levels are above 40 micrograms/dL. There are $28 million in emergency funds provided for this crisis. The hope was that some could be earmarked for pasteurized donor milk.

Literature describing the attributes of a good wet nurse dates back as far as 2250 BC, but the notion of systematically donating expressed milk wasn't highlighted until 1934. Likely the most famous case of mothers donating their milk to saves lives was when the Dionne quintuplets were born in northern Ontario. These identical girls were born at home, where there was no running water or electricity. The mother, who had birthed six babies prior to this pregnancy thought she "might" be having twins. The babies arrived 8 weeks early with a total weight of 13 pounds 5 ounces. The birth was attended by a physician and two midwives. A nurse caring for the children went about the area, and by their 52nd hour of life, she was able to secure two ounces of milk from women who were lactating. Within four days, a newborn specialist physician shipped an incubator and donor milk. Word of the need traveled fast in Canada, and the Toronto Junior League began to receive and ship donated milk by train. In the 4 months they were given human milk, women had donated over 8,000 ounces to keep Yvonne, Marie, Emilie, Annette, and Cecile alive. It's an amazing story and one that is repeated every day in all corners of America and beyond.

Chapter Nineteen

EDUCATING THE NEXT GENERATION OF PEDIATRICIANS

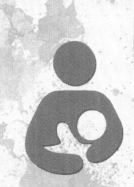

Bookends

Between the intern's ears
are thousands of pieces
of medical information,
lighting up in their brains
when called upon by professors,
like the motion sensor of a home—
light illuminating darkness.

How best to spend 60 minutes
of lecture with every new group—
each month, is its own challenge.
Always one sleepy doc trying to
stay awake for 32 hours,
his final hour post-call, until
regulations put an ended to that insanity.

July intern, fresh out of med school—
eager, wide-eyed, same intern twelve months

later, often less receptive.
Women docs usually more interested,
especially if they've had a pregnancy—
or a breastfeeding experience.
Men, less so, save the dad of a breastfed child.

Indeed, there are important studies,
facts, and numbers to discuss
in the field of lactation,
but these can be memorized
in a matter of minutes.
What do I impart that will make
a lasting impression?

Whatever their disposition,
they respond to stories,
the faces, triumphs, and tragedies
that make the science matter—
why close follow-up after discharge
is so critical, or the importance
of weights and breast exams.

They know my son
has one kidney,
discovered on a fluke
when he was 22,
that human milk
was less stress
on that sole kidney.

His brother,
with multiple ear infections
as a child,

reminds that mother's milk
is no panacea,
lowering disease risk–
not eliminating.

They know my daughter,
two days after giving birth declared
Breastfeeding sucks, mom.
Unlike so many who would
have weaned, she made it through,
admonishing, should I repeat that story,
I tell of the treasure breastfeeding became.

They know my oldest earned a PhD,
that medium-chain
fatty acids in human milk
contribute to brain growth,
that early IQ studies accounted for
demographic confounders
associated with higher IQ.

Coupled with my own stories,
I tell the sagas
of first-time moms
trying to put newborns on
unrealistic feeding schedules,
or misunderstood phone instructions
that resulted in rehospitalizations.

The stories
connect the dots.
They translate book-knowledge
to real journeys of patients–

from recommendations
of the health care provider to
outcomes for the baby.

They appreciate.
They empathize.
They begin to understand,
drawn in by the story,
repercussions–
imprinted in the space
between their ears.

In 1976, my career began
with a witty and compassionate
resident in pediatric intensive care.
In 2015, my final year of lectures
ended with his intern-daughter–
serendipitous bookends
to resident education.

Chapter Twenty

REFLECTIONS WHILE ON LEAVE

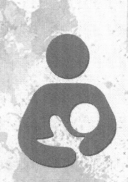

Faces of Diversity

*In each of our interactions we begin to
realize there is something benevolent in
the other that helps us let down our
defenses and defensiveness.*

RICHARD ROHR

IMMORTAL DIAMOND

It's the 29th of February, that odd relative that only comes around once in a while. The ground hog didn't see his shadow at the beginning of the month, and I am taking a walk in only a lightweight jacket. It's wonderful weather here in Southern Ohio.

A county park is two blocks from the home where I've lived a little over 10 years. I walk here three or four times a week.

On weekdays, there may only be a few people walking or running
the loop around the lake, but on the weekends, as the weather
warms, it can look like an Easter parade—steady streams of adults,
kids, and pets. There has always been a pretty even racial mix
on the trail, even before Michelle Obama launched her school
fitness campaign, *Let's Move*. On Saturday mornings, I often see
a team from a local Black church, men and women who look to
be in their 40s, 50s, and 60s, wearing t-shirts with their church
logo. I enjoy seeing the comradery and overhearing their banter
even above the sound of the book tape I'm listening to with
headphones.

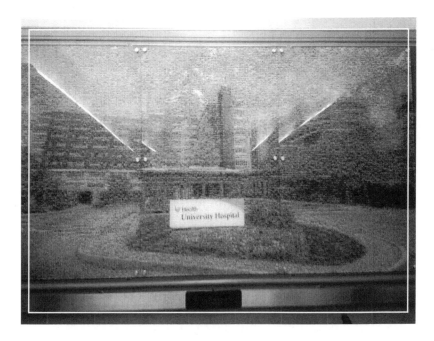

∗ Collage of UCMC/UC Health employees ∗

In the last couple of years, there have been more Hispanics,
running, or walking alone, as couples, with friends, or with children.

The diversity reflects the growing diversity in Cincinnati: 46% African American, 48% White, 2% Asian, 3% Hispanic (which may not be capturing undocumented immigrants), and 1.29% other. It's this 1.29% that piques my interest today.

I am walking up the back loop away from the lake and hear music—percussion, reed, and flute. I recognize it as Arabic in origin, even before I see seven or eight Muslim women covered in their colorful hijabs. Even though they are at a distant set of picnic tables, they are atop a hill, so I can easily see they are greeting each other with an embrace and kiss on each cheek while the children run in and around them. I'm distracted away from my book tape. If there is any community, any area where they are safe, it should be here in this county park where diversity is embraced. Yet still, I worry. The awareness of the worry saddens me.

As I make my way downhill toward the lake again, there are two younger Muslim women, one with hijab in hand, one wearing her garb. The traditionally dressed woman is taking photos of the other with her smart phone. Her hair is blowing in the wind and she has a wide smile across her face. I wonder. Which is safer, standing out by wearing the hijab or melting in like everyone else? I don't have an answer, and maybe it's not even the right question.

As I finish up my walk, I stop by the public restrooms. There is a mother and her toddler daughter. I see the toddler first and she blends in like any other toddler. I look up and see her mother in the more conservative Muslim garb, the burqa, with only a moon sliver of open garment for her eyes to meet mine.

This woman and any of the others could have been prior patients of mine. Yet, in the hospital, surrounded by IVs and blood pressure cuffs, and even with the hijab, all women seem very much the same. I take time to ask and read about the countries of my patients. I hear much on the news too. I'm well aware and deeply troubled by the Taliban in Afghanistan, Boca Haram in northeast Nigeria, ISIS in Syria and beyond, Al Qaeda in Pakistan, Al-Shabab in Kenya and Somalia, and domestic terrorists and thugs at home and abroad. But the vast majority of people here and elsewhere are not radicals and in my hospital, they are simply new mothers and dads. I love the bumper sticker with the varied symbols of religions that simply says "Co-exist." That is my prayer.

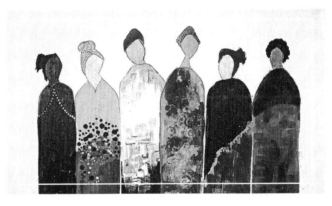

✶ Iconic Cross- Cultural Mural,
Artist Unknown ✶

Six months later, I am making this same trip around the lake when, even with my headphones on, I catch a conversation of two African American moms as they stroll their babies. After passing, I turn around and holler *Excuse Me*, and they turn and pause.

"Were you talking about difficulties with breastfeeding?"

"Yes!!"

"I have my own family member struggling now too. How old are your babies?"

"One month."

"Wow, same age as my granddaughter! I'm also a breastfeeding consultant at University. But even so, it's hard to help a relative when you don't live with them."

"Yeah, I've been reading. I think she's just clustering feedings at night. I'm so tired in the morning."

Her friend chimes in, "She's doing better than me. I'm doing more pumping now."

We chat about the challenges of new motherhood, and the joys, and I run into them again when the babies are 2 months and 3-and-a-half months old. They give me an update on their babies. They're hanging in with breastfeeding. One of them is reading a book about how the French raise children, and has gotten some good tips on helping her baby sleep better at night. On this walk, I'm strolling my granddaughter and we each peer into one another's strollers to see our bundles of joy.

Chapter Twenty-One

AFTERWARD

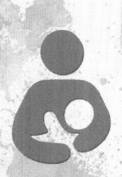

Passing the Torch

*What is the meaning of life? To humbly and
proudly return what you've been given.*

UNKNOWN

My work has seen me through six remodels of the lobby,
several chief nursing officers, and five name changes. We are
now the University of Cincinnati Medical Center. The lobby's
high ceilings, pools of water, plants, and lovely courtyard give
it the ambience of a grand hotel. I've seen the seasons of my
life pass here, as well, like the changing colors, plants, and
flowers blooming in the courtyard garden. It's the patients
themselves who ultimately draw me back here. Most are not
rich by society's standards, but they have a wealth of stories
in their bodies, minds, and hearts. And I, I have more to learn

from them. It is well worth the strange experience of a nurse standing guard outside the bathroom of Personnel Health during my "pre-employment" appointment, as I pee into a blue toilet bowl that somehow assures them that I've not cheated on the urine drug screen I am taking. It must be how it goes regularly for our moms in their drug treatment centers, as they try to stay on the wagon and provide their random urine samples.

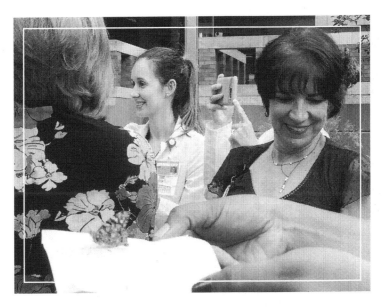

✳ *World Breastfeeding Week Celebration and Butterfly Release* ✳

My work is infrequent enough now that I don't take on big projects that keep me late and keep Ron up worrying about me. Even without the projects, it's enough to enjoy encounters with moms and babies, and focus on the immediacy of what their needs require. The program continues to expand, and I am so thankful that the work continues with others carrying the torch, leading the way, and bearing the burdens of program development that are no longer mine. It is a privileged place to be. In August 2017, we celebrated World Breastfeeding Month with staff and invited guests. During the ceremony, the department was presented with a $47,000 check. The grant is supporting our ability to provide after-hours phone support to mothers in 18 of Ohio's counties. The event closed with a lovely butterfly release in the courtyard.

There have been 19 LCs employed by the hospital's lactation department over a 25-year period. Nine are currently employed. Four are full-time (though one works almost completely in another capacity), two are part-time, and three work a very intermittent status (PRN). All of them, in one way or another, have helped me, both through the day-to-day rubbing of shoulders, and through the sharing of knowledge and experience, to grow personally and professionally. I want to acknowledge a special few. Joan, who, though not an IBCLC, filling in for me during the Pilot Project; Nancy, who worked tirelessly for the moms and put up with me leaving her lengthy, detailed notes on dozens of small post-it pads; Krista, who added humor and computer skills to make our department more professional and who *had me at hello* during her interview when she said she had a passion for breastfeeding; June, gifted educator and innovator; and finally, Sue, to whom I happily passed down the mantle of leadership for the department in 2010. She has exercised every quality of a good leader and I am proud to call her friend. In addition, she pays attention to detail (a bit of my opposite there), but so essential to carry us through the Baby-Friendly certification and its ongoing responsibilities. And though not a lactation consultant, our manager, Ruby, exuded the leadership, savvy, and bold vision, to carry Women's Health Services through the process to become Baby-Friendly. I, we, owe her an unpayable debt of gratitude.

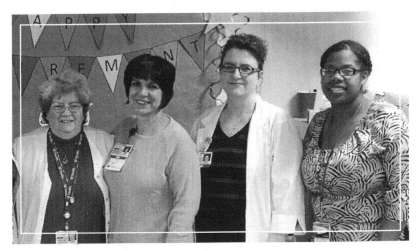

*Past & Present LC team: Helen, Sue, June,
and Cierra, our WIC peer counselor* *

* Nancy, IBCLC *

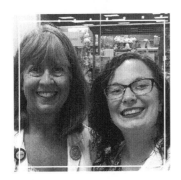

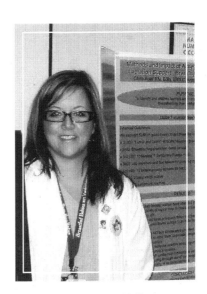

Chris with Brandi, IBCLC   * Krista, IBCLC *

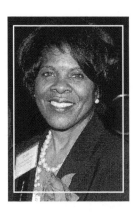 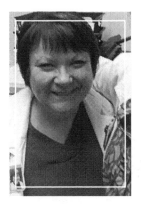

*Ruby Crawford-Hemphill,
Assistant Chief Nursing
Officer*

Olga, IBCLC

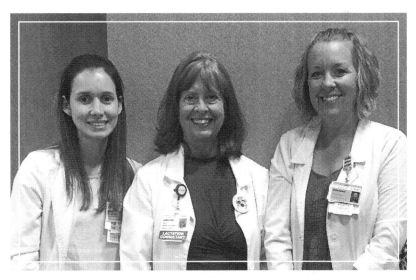

Laia, Chris, Stephanie, IBCLC's

I have received practice in Spanish from Olga and Laia, had support through a difficult time from Gail, learned awesome approaches to parent education and effective communication from Robin, appreciated the work that Stephanie has put into developing our outpatient program, laughed with Kim about the short-lived LC who always gagged on colostrum, enjoyed mentoring Tashia, and thoroughly enjoyed Brandi's youthful zeal. When a new lactation consultant tells me, "I have a passion for breastfeeding," that's all I need to hear to know that she is trainable and worthy of taking up the torch to carry the department professionally and compassionately, into the future. All will be safe.

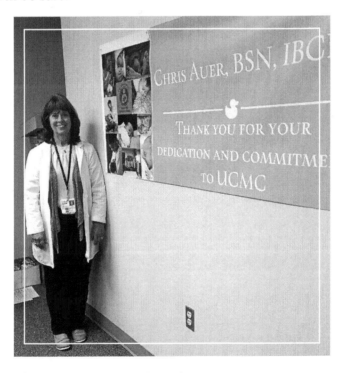

✳ Retirement ✳

But the sum of the individual parts does not make the stool of quality breastfeeding support and patient care stay upright. It's the three legs of shared values, strong leadership from management, and buy-in from the boots-on-the-ground staff, that stabilize the stool. The shared values are embodied in the Ten Steps implemented with good assessment and compassionate care. They include:

» Developing policies to guide care,
» Teaching them to the staff to assure implementation,
» Educating mothers prenatally so their feeding decision, regardless of what it is, will be supported because it is based on understanding the value of human milk and the risks associated with other choices,
» Placing all babies skin-to-skin against their mother's chest immediately after birth (and through the first breastfeeding for those who opt to nurse),
» Assisting mothers with nursing and/or pumping should they be separated from their baby,
» Supporting exclusive breastfeeding as recommended by the American Academy of Pediatrics, unless a medical necessity arises,
» Promoting non-separation of mothers and babies,
» Encouraging feeding on the basis of cues, not the clock,
» Avoiding bottles and pacifiers while breastfeeding is being established, and
» Referring mothers to support systems after discharge from the hospital.

I read the steps now and they seem so obvious. Yet, they require diligent attention in order for breastfeeding mothers to receive the care they need and deserve. Still, their needs are always beyond breastfeeding, even beyond acquiring the role of parent. I have learned this, and so much more from them. I hope I have met them where they are, received them, listened to their stories, looked into their eyes, and served them—body, mind, and spirit.

This is what you shall do; Love the earth and sun and the animals, despise riches, give alms to everyone that asks, stand up for the stupid and crazy, devote your income and labor to others, hate tyrants, argue not concerning God, have patience and indulgence toward the people, take off your hat to nothing known or unknown or to any man or number of men, go freely with powerful uneducated persons and with the young and with the mothers of families, read these leaves in the open air every season of every year of your life, re-examine all you have been told at school or church or in any book, dismiss whatever insults your own soul, and your very flesh shall be a great poem and have the richest fluency not only in its words but in the silent lines of its lips and face and between the lashes of your eyes and in every motion and joint of your body.

WALT WHITMAN

About the Author

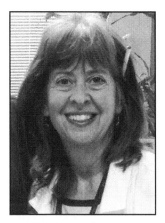

Chris Auer has spent the last forty years assisting and listening to mothers, fathers, families, and health care providers at the University of Cincinnati Medical Center. No matter the nationality, race, or income level, a mother and father are vulnerable in the early days and weeks following birth. With a commitment to holistic care, she has worked passionately to companion mothers and families on this segment of their life journey. In the retelling of their stories, we see the importance of meeting others where they are *in the moment*, with a respectful acceptance and caring, listening presence.

For twenty-five years Chris provided a monthly breastfeeding lecture to pediatric residents and mentored lactation interns, combining research –based information with an emphasis on compassionate listening, empowering each mother to make her own decision as she navigates the early period of parenting. Chris has published in scientific journals on topics ranging from evidence-based practice to breastfeeding quadruplets, from ankyloglossia to donor milk and quality improvement projects for very-low birth weight infants. The sharing of these poignant encounters surrounding birth, breastfeeding, and the life circumstances of families from over seventy-seven countries is her first published exploration of the personal dimension of working with families and staff. She is also a wife, mother to four adult children, grandmother of four, and spiritual companion to friends in her faith community in Spring Grove Village, Cincinnati, Ohio. Each of these, her personal connections, has in turn influenced her own perspective and journey.

You Might Also Like

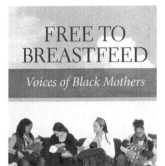

Free to Breastfeed: Voices of Black Mothers

Jeanine Valrie Logan
Anaya Sangodele-Ayoka

Free to Breastfeed: Voices from Black Mothers outpaces other books on the topic because it gives privilege to actual women. Facts about breastfeeding and statistics can be found in numerous pamphlets and with professional lactation consultants. However, there is no other book on the market that can give a new or expectant mother the experience of seeing her experience reflected in the stories and pictures of other women. While there is growing coverage to the disparities in breastfeeding rates, the actual thoughts and experiences of African-American nursing mothers are overlooked. It is precisely these first-hand experiences that breastfeeding mothers seek from other women.

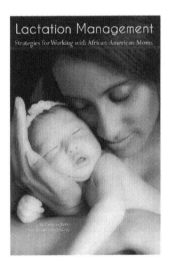

Lactation Management: Strategies for Working with African-American Moms

Katherine Barber

Do you need help promoting breastfeeding to your African-American clients? Katherine Barber, founder of the African American Breastfeeding Alliance and author of The Black Woman's Guide to Breastfeeding, shares her experience and knowledge with you in *Lactation Management: Strategies for Working with African-American Moms*

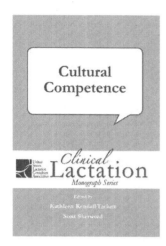

Clinical Lactation Monograph Series: Cultural Competence

Edited by
Kathleen Kendall-Tackett
Scott Sherwood

Cultural Competency is a concise collection of articles that will help you improve your effectiveness when working with mothers from different cultures. Topics include:

• Assumptions about different cultural groups and how they impact breastfeeding support

• Shoshone and Arapaho tribal breastfeeding traditions shared through oral folklore

• Barriers to decreasing health disparities in infant mortality for African Americans

• Effects of inflammation and trauma on health disparities that result in higher rates of infant mortality among minority populations

• Barriers to breastfeeding experienced by Black mothers and how lactation consultants can support them more effectively

• Social support and breastfeeding self-efficacy among Black mothers

• Decreasing pregnancy, birth, and lactation health disparities in the urban core

• Positive changes in breastfeeding rates within the African American community

• Grassroots breastfeeding organizations serving African American mothers

Made in the USA
Middletown, DE
17 March 2018